Alzheimer's Disease: Clinical and Treatment Perspectives

This publication was made possible by a grant from the Neuroscience Unit of Hoechst-Roussel Pharmaceuticals, Inc.

Alzheimer's Disease: Clinical and Treatment Perspectives

Edited by

N. R. CUTLER
California Clinical Trials, Beverly Hills, California, USA

C. G. GOTTFRIES
Department of Clinical Neuroscience, University of Göteborg, Sweden

K. SIEGFRIED
Clinical Research Department, Hoechst AG, Frankfurt, Germany

JOHN WILEY & SONS

Chichester · New York · Brisbane · Toronto · Singapore

Baffins Lane, Chichester,
West Sussex PO19 1UD, England
Telephone: National Chichester (0243) 779777
International +44 243 779777

Reprinted November 1995 and September 1996

Other Wiley Editorial Offices

John Wiley & Sons, Inc., 605 Third Avenue,
New York, NY 10158-0012, USA

Jacaranda Wiley Ltd, 33 Park Road, Milton,
Queensland 4064, Australia

John Wiley & Sons (Canada) Ltd, 22 Worcester Road,
Rexdale, Ontario M9W 1L1, Canada

John Wiley & Sons (SEA) Pte Ltd, 37 Jalan Pemimpin #05-04,
Block B, Union Industrial Building, Singapore 2057

Library of Congress Cataloging-in-Publication Data

Alzheimer's disease : clinical and treatment perspectives / edited by
N.R. Cutler, C.G. Gottfries, and K.R. Siegfried.
p. cm.
Includes bibliographical references and index.
ISBN 0 471 95039 4
1. Alzheimer's disease—Pathophysiology. 2. Alzheimer's disease—
treatment. I. Cutler, Neal R. II. Gottfries, C.G.
III. Siegfried, Klaudius, 1948–
[DNLM: 1. Alzheimer's Disease. WM 220 A4778208 1994]
RC523.A3964 1994
616.85'23–dc20
DNLM/DLC
for Library of Congress 94–22396
CIP

British Library Cataloguing in Publication Data

A catalogue record for this book is available
from the British Library

ISBN 0 471 95039 4

Typeset in 11/13 pt Palatino by Dorwyn Ltd
Printed and bound in Great Britain by
Biddles Ltd, Guildford and King's Lynn

Contents

Contributors

Dr Kaj Blennow, Göteborg University, Department of Clinical Neuroscience, Mölndal Hospital, Mölndal, Sweden

Dr David M. Bowen, Institute of Neurology, Miriam Marks Department of Neurobiology, London, UK

Dr Christopher P. L-H. Chen, Miriam Marks Department of Neurochemistry, Institute of Neurology, Queen Square, London; and Department of Neuropathology, Radcliffe Infirmary, Oxford, UK

Dr. Iain P. Chessel, Miriam Marks Department of Neurochemistry, Institute of Neurology, Queen Square, London, UK

Dr Alan J. Cross, Astra Neuroscience Research Unit, London, UK

Dr Neal R. Cutler, California Clinical Trials, Beverly Hills, CA, USA

Dr Richard C. Effland, Department of Chemical Research, Neuroscience Strategic Business Unit, Hoechst-Roussel Pharmaceuticals, Inc., Somerville, NJ, USA

Dr Paul T. Francis, Miriam Marks Department of Neurochemistry, Institute of Neurology, Queen Square, London, UK

Dr Carl-Gerhard Gottfries, Göteborg University, Department of Clinical Neuroscience, Mölndal Hospital, Mölndal, Sweden

Dr Johan Gottfries, Göteborg University, Department of Clinical Neuroscience, Mölndal Hospital, Mölndol, Sweden

Dr A. Richard Green, Astra Neuroscience Research Unit, London, UK

Dr Francis J. Huff, Clinical Neuroscience, Hoechst-Roussel Pharmaceuticals Inc., Somerville, NJ, USA

Dr Ingrar Karlsson, Göteborg University, Department of Clinical Neuroscience, Mölndal Hospital, Mölndal, Sweden

Dr Lawrence L. Martin, Department of Chemical Research, Neuroscience Strategic Business Unit, Hoechst-Roussel Pharmaceuticals, Inc., Somerville, NJ, USA

Dr Michael F. Murphy, Cephalon, Inc., West Chester, PA, USA

Dr David Neary, Department of Neurology, Manchester Royal Infirmary, Manchester, UK

Dr Andrew W. Procter, Miriam Marks Department of Neurochemistry, Institute of Neurology, Queen Square, London, UK; and Department of Psychiatry, United Medical and Dental Schools (Guy's Campus), London, UK

Dr Michelle Qume, Miriam Marks Department of Neurochemistry, Institute of Neurology, Queen Square, London, UK

Dr Garth E. Ringheim, Department of Biological Research, Neuroscience Strategic Business Unit, Hoechst-Roussel Pharmaceuticals, Inc., Somerville, NJ, USA

Dr Sudhir R. Sahasrabudhe, Department of Molecular Neurobiology, Neuroscience Strategic Business Unit, Hoechst-Roussel Pharmaceuticals, Inc., Somerville, NJ, USA

Dr Philip Scheltens, Vakgroep Neurologie, Academisch Ziekenhuis der Vrije Universiteit, Amsterdam, The Netherlands

Dr Klaudius Siegfried, Clinical Research Department, H-840, Hoechst AG, Frankfurt am Main, Germany

Dr John J. Sramek, California Clinical Trials, Beverly Hills, California, USA

Dr L. Svennerholm, Department of Psychiatry and Neurochemistry, Mölndal, Sweden

Dr Anders Wallin, Department of Clinical Neuroscience, Section of Psychiatry and Neurochemistry, University of Göteborg, Mölndal Hospital, Mölndal, Sweden

Dr Marie-Thérèse Webster, Miriam Marks Department of Neurochemistry, Institute of Neurology, Queen Square, London, UK

Dr Carole Wilmot, Neuroscience Strategic Business Unit, Hoechst-Roussel Pharmaceuticals Inc., Somerville, NJ, USA

Preface

Though the treatment of Alzheimer's disease (AD) presents a great challenge to neuroscience research, progress in recent years has been substantial. A clearer picture of the disease process has emerged, prompting a diverse array of investigations. While much attention has been focused on developing drugs which restore neurotransmitter deficits, particularly those associated with the loss of cholinergic neurons seen in AD, other approaches are also being explored. Nootropics, CNS stimulants, and vasodilators have been examined as alternative symptomatic treatments, and new therapeutic strategies targeted at the pathophysiology of AD, including interventions in amyloid plaque formation, immune-mediated mechanisms and free radical-induced brain pathology, attempt to retard or completely halt disease progression. Many of these approaches are discussed here. Another important branch of research covered in this volume is the identification of *in vivo* biochemical markers that may help to differentiate among various types of AD and other dementia disorders. Such markers may permit earlier diagnosis—and thus treatment—of AD, and would make clinical trial results more relevant to individual disease pathologies by providing a mechanism to easily identify subjects who share the same type of dementia. A third component of AD research employs creative and efficient methodologies to facilitate development of potential compounds for the treatment of AD; for example, this volume concludes by describing an innovative protocol termed a 'bridging study' that expedites the drug development process by enrolling AD patients into phase I multiple-dose safety/tolerance studies in order to ultimately determine an optimal dosage for use in phase II/III efficacy studies.

N.R. Cutler, C.G. Gottfries and K. Siegfried, October 1994

1

The Diagnosis of Alzheimer's Disease

C. G. Gottfries, K. Blennow, J. Gottfries, I. Karlsson, and A. Wallin

Department of Clinical Neuroscience, University of Göteborg, Mölndal, Sweden

ABSTRACT

Since the seventies, the original rare form of Alzheimer's disease (AD) and senile dementia of the Alzheimer type (SDAT) have been sampled as one group because of an assumed similar clinical phenomenology and the presence of Alzheimer brain lesions (senile plaques and neurofibrillary tangles) in both disorders. A significant correlation between Alzheimer lesions and cognitive disturbances also supported this sampling. However, none of the reasons for combining the two disorders are valid. A careful investigation of the symptomatology has shown that symptoms indicating parieto-temporal lobe disturbances predominate in early-onset AD, whereas a more general symptomatology prevails in SDAT. Confusional symptoms and leukoaraiosis also significantly differentiate the two disorders, as do some biological markers, e.g. ganglioside and chromogranin A concentrations in CSF. Postmortem studies also indicate gray-matter

Alzheimer's Disease: Clinical and Treatment Perspectives. Edited by N. R. Cutler, C. G. Gottfries and K. Siegfried.

membrane disturbances in AD, whereas disturbances of myelin components are more evident in SDAT.

Calculations were made on a data set of 29 descriptor variables where the data were fitted to a partial least squares discriminant analysis (PLS) model. The statistical analysis showed that the subgrouping carried out on consecutive dementia patients was genuine and that three subgroups emerged: vascular dementia, SDAT, and AD. According to the data, AD patients appear to be a relatively homogeneous group, while the group of SDAT patients is more scattered and evidently less homogeneous. There is a great need for improved diagnostic methodology concerning dementia of the Alzheimer type.

INTRODUCTION

When Alzheimer in 1906 first described 'a characteristic disease of the cerebral cortex', he had a 51-year-old woman in mind. Kraepelin (1910) in the paper 'Senile and Presenile Dementias' created the concept of Alzheimer's disease and in his paper he states:

> While the anatomical findings suggest that we are dealing with a particularly serious form of senile dementia, the fact that this disease sometimes starts already around the age of 40 does not allow this supposition. In such cases we should at least assume a 'senium praecox', if not perhaps a more or less age-independent unique disease process.

According to the epidemiological and familial investigations by Sjögren *et al.* (1952), Larsson *et al.* (1963) and Sourander and Sjögren (1970), the presenile form of Alzheimer's disease (AD) and senile dementia behave as two different disorders. There is a fourfold increased risk of senile dementia in siblings of senile demented patients. No instances of AD were found in the 2675 family members investigated. Heston *et al.* (1981) found that relatives of AD patients ran a markedly increased risk of getting AD.

As neuropathologists have found Alzheimer lesions, e.g. senile plaques (SPs) and neurofibrillary tangles (NFPs), also in brains from patients with late onset dementia, the latter form has been called senile dementia of the Alzheimer type (SDAT). Especially in the United States, the two forms of Alzheimer dementia have been sampled as one (AD/SDAT). The main reasons for combining AD and SDAT are as follows:

- Similar clinical phenomenology.
- Alzheimer lesions are present in both disorders.
- There are significant correlations between Alzheimer lesions and behavioral disturbances.

None of these reasons for combining the two disorders are valid. Before sampling two disorders as one, it should be verified that they have identical etiology/pathology and clinical course.

CLINICAL DIAGNOSIS

The criteria outlined by the American Psychiatric Association (APA) in the *Diagnostic and Statistical Manual of Mental Disorders* have been generally accepted for diagnosis of dementia. Compulsory criteria for dementia in the revised version (DSM-III-R) are:

1. Memory impairment.
2. At least one of the following disturbances:
   a. Impaired abstract thinking
   b. Impaired judgement
   c. Aphasia, apraxia, agnosia or constructional difficulties
   d. Personality change
3. The disturbance above interferes significantly with work and/or social activities or relations.
4. The disturbance does not occur exclusively during the course of delirium.
5. Evidence from the history, physical examination or laboratory tests of a specific organic factor.

For the clinical diagnosis of AD/SDAT, there are two major diagnostic manuals, the NINCDS-ADRDA criteria (McKhann *et al.*, 1984) and the DSM-III-R. These two manuals are compatible. The NINCDS-ADRDA criteria include:

1. The presence of progressive dementia with deficits in two or more areas of cognition.

2. No disturbance of consciousness at the time of diagnosis.
3. Onset between ages 40 and 90.
4. Absence of systemic disorders or other brain diseases, e.g. multi-infarct dementia and depression, that could account for the deficits.

The DSM-III-R criteria for AD/SDAT include:

1. The presence of progressive dementia with a multifaceted loss of intellectual abilities.
2. The exclusion of all other possible causes of the dementia.

It is obvious that the above criteria are, in fact, exclusion criteria and, therefore, the diagnosis of 'probable' AD/SDAT is made.

The definite diagnosis of AD/SDAT is made postmortem after histopathological investigation of the brain. A major part of the scientific work on AD/SDAT has been based on NFPs and SPs, although their relation to the etiology and pathogenesis of AD is unknown. It is still an open question whether these neuropathological findings are primary phenomena or only of a secondary nature, unrelated to the etiology of the disease. In recent years, it has become more and more clear that NFTs and SPs cannot be considered the golden standards for diagnosis, as they are found in a variety of disorders: postencephalitic Parkinson's disease, the Guam Parkinson dementia complex, dementia pugilistica, mental retardation due to Down's syndrome or other causes, subacute sclerosing panencephalitis, Creutzfeldt-Jakob disease, chronic tuberculosis, lead and magnesium poisoning, progressive supranuclear palsy, and tuberous sclerosis. At present, neuropathologists also assume that the diagnosis of AD/SDAT should be made by studying not only the presence of SPs and NFTs, but also degeneration of synapses, formation of amyloid, and membrane disturbances.

ONE STEP BACK

As the clinical diagnosis of AD/SDAT is an exclusion diagnosis, and as the postmortem diagnosis of AD/SDAT is nonspecific, the time has come to take one step back. The question is whether we should go back to the subgrouping suggested by Kraepelin and Sjögren and Sourander, i.e., to divide Alzheimer-type dementia into an early-onset form, AD, and a late-onset form, SDAT, considering them two disorders.

POSTMORTEM HETEROGENEITY

As is evident from postmortem findings (this volume, Chapter 5), there are not only quantitative but also qualitative differences between early-onset AD and SDAT concerning concentrations of membrane components. According to this study, AD is a cortical disease, whereas SDAT is a disorder that mostly damages white matter.

CLINICAL HETEROGENEITY

In a study by Blennow and Wallin (1992), the symptomatology of AD/SDAT was investigated. This topic is of interest, because there is an inconsistency between the literature and contemporary diagnostic manuals. AD/SDAT is proposed to have a characteristic symptomatology of memory disturbances and cortical symptoms of parietal type, whereas, according to the diagnostic manuals, AD/SDAT should be diagnosed by way of exclusion, irrespective of the symptomatology. The study revealed two subgroups, one with predominant cortical symptoms of parietal type (AD early onset) and another with general cognitive symptoms but absence of or only mild cortical symptoms (SDAT). In AD, the age at onset was significantly lower, confusional symptoms and leukoaraiosis on computerized tomographic scans were less frequent, and the ganglioside GM1 concentration in cerebrospinal fluid was significantly higher than in SDAT. According to the authors, the relation between symptomatology and leukoaraiosis suggests that leukoaraiosis has clinical significance in AD/SDAT.

In clinical studies of patients with AD/SDAT at our department, 20 patients with AD, 34 patients with SDAT and 12 patients with vascular dementia (VAD) were clinically investigated. Medical history, physical, neurological and psychiatric examination, screening laboratory tests, ECG, X-ray of the chest, EEG and computerized tomography (CT) of the brain were performed. The data set consisted of 29 descriptor variables, including clinical chemistry, duration of disease, degree of brain lesions, and infarction status, etc. The information about age at onset of disease and age at entering the study were not included in the descriptor variable set. Calculations were made using the SIMCA 4.4 software package (Umetri, Umeå, Sweden) and the data were fitted to a PLS model (Höskuldsson, 1988) using dummy variables for the response variables (the clinical diagnoses). The descriptor variables are described in Table 1. The only variables significantly separating AD and SDAT were the presence of parietal symptomatology and nonregional symptomatology (Table 1). The variance of some descriptor variables could not be accounted for by the PLS model, as they had less than 5% of their total variance explained. The blood pressure variables were in a range from 3 to 10%, while the other variables had 15–65% of their total variance explained. Cross validation showed that, if patients with only mild symptoms were excluded, the diagnose variables had 68–72% of their total variance explained. The data showed that the subgrouping of consecutive dementia patients was genuine, and this was evident despite the deliberate removal of any variable containing information about age or age at onset of disease. (The inclusion of age variables would presumably add further strength to the present classification.) As is evident from Figure 1, the classification of the three diagnoses contained some overlap. It is also evident from the figure that the VAD and AD groups did not overlap and should be easy to divide clinically. Between SDAT and the two other forms overlap appears to occur. It is obvious that an AD patient might be 65 years or a few years older at onset of disease and an SDAT patient could already suffer from clear symptoms at an age below 65. This was obvious from the family studies by Larsson *et al.* (1963), as well as from the clinical study by Blennow and Wallin (1992). Between VAD and SDAT, a slightly different pattern of overlap is depicted, including a gray zone. Patients in this zone might be misclassified, but it is more probable that they suffer from both SDAT and VAD. As is evident from Figure 2, in which only AD and SDAT patients are depicted, AD appears to be a relatively homogeneous group, whereas the SDAT patients are more scattered and evidently less homogeneous.

Table 1 *Means and standard deviations of the descriptor variables in the diagnostic groups*

	AD (n=20)		VAD (n=12)		SDAT (n=34)	
	Mean	SD	Mean	SD	Mean	SD
Albumin ratio	6.02*	1.63	10.35	4.46	7.34	2.82
Bilateral pyramidal signs	0.40	0.50	0.42	0.51	0.09	0.29
Bilateral extrapyramidal signs	0.05	0.22	0.50	0.52	0.15	0.36
Central lacunas	0.10	0.31	0.42	0.51	0.21	0.41
Central atrophy	1.20	0.89	1.83	0.72	1.35	0.95
Confusional symptoms	0.00*	0.00	0.42	0.51	0.65	0.69
Cortical infarcts	0.00	0.00	0.33	0.49	0.00	0.00
Cortical atrophy	1.75	0.72	2.00	0.60	1.76	0.74
CSF-5-HIAA	115.10	43.10	109.92	29.08	124.59	48.54
CSF-HMPG	41.65	6.51	43.08	9.88	47.03	17.99
CSF-HVA	219.00	100.38	191.08	89.41	212.50	94.57
Diabetes mellitus	0.00*	0.00	40.50	0.52	0.06	0.24
Duration	5.45	2.11	4.50	1.45	4.06	2.33
Focal pyramidal signs	0.00*	0.00	0.50	0.52	0.06	0.24
Frontal symptoms	0.65	0.59	1.00	0.43	0.35	0.49
Hypertension	0.20	0.41	0.58	0.51	0.24	0.43
IgG index	0.50	0.18	0.52	0.07	0.49	0.18
Ischemic heart disease	0.20	0.41	0.58	0.51	0.41	0.50
Lying diastolic blood pressure	80.70	11.59	82.09	10.98	81.73	10.88
Lying systolic blood pressure	139.30	22.52	146.82	22.78	150.18	20.57
Nonregional symptoms	0.25	0.44	0.42	0.51	0.85†	0.36
Parietal symptoms	1.45*	0.69	0.33	0.65	0.35†	0.69
Pseudobulbar signs	0.00*	0.00	0.42	0.51	0.03	0.17
Severity of dementia	1.75	0.72	1.92	0.67	1.41	0.50
Sex	1.45	0.51	1.33	0.49	1.74	0.45
Subcortical symptoms	0.30*	0.47	1.33	0.65	0.21‡	0.41
Vascular disease	0.30*	0.47	1.00	0.00	0.53	0.51
White matter lesions—extension	0.40*	0.82	1.92	1.08	1.21	0.88
White matter lesions—intensity	0.40*	0.82	1.92	1.08	1.21	0.88

* $p<0.05$ univariate analysis for differences between AD and VAD.
† $p<$ univariate analysis for differences between AD and SDAT.
‡ $p<$ univariate analysis for differences between VAD and SDAT.

IMPROVEMENT OF DIAGNOSIS

As is obvious from the study by Blennow and Wallin (1992) and from the presentation by Blennow (this volume, Chapter 2), it is worth while searching for biochemical markers for subgroups of

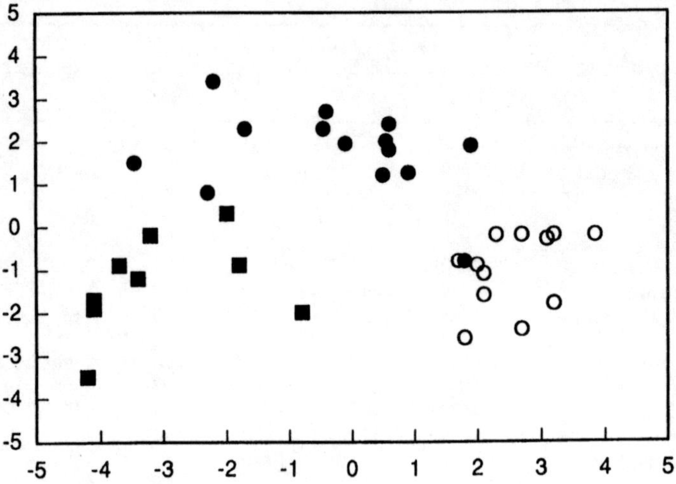

Figure 1 *The distribution of patients with Alzheimer's disease (AD) early onset (○), with senile dementia of the Alzheimer type (SDAT) late onset (●) and vascular dementia (■) according to 29 descriptor variables. Calculations made using the SIMCA 4.4 software package*

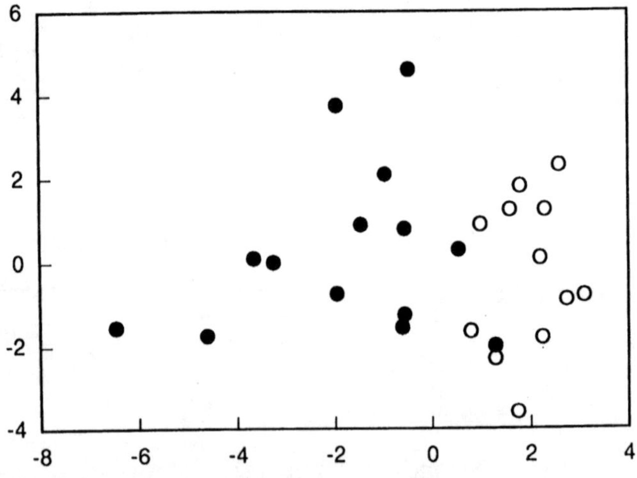

Figure 2 *The distribution of patients with Alzheimer's disease (AD) early onset (○) and with senile dementia of the Alzheimer type (SDAT) late onset (●) according to 29 descriptor variables. Calculations made using the SIMCA 4.4 software package*

dementia included in the present concept of AD/SDAT. Evidently, brain imaging techniques must also be used in the search for homogeneous subgroups of dementia within the group of AD/SDAT (this volume, Chapter 3). In some studies, peripheral markers have also been used in the efforts to separate homogeneous subgroups of disorders within AD/SDAT. In a study by Regland *et al.* (1988), it was obvious that around 23% of patients with AD/SDAT have low vitamin B12 levels without having anemia. In other studies by the same group of investigators, it was shown that a selective vitamin B12 deficiency in CNS might be present in patients with dementia disorders. Basun (1993) showed that the metabolism of several trace elements and heavy metals are disturbed in patients with AD/SDAT. Landin *et al.* (1993) showed that patients with dementia disorders can be divided into subgroups with respectively, a hypermetabolic and a hypometabolic syndrome. This division might also be used in the separation of homogeneous subgroups.

SUGGESTED SUBGROUPS OF ALZHEIMER-TYPE DEMENTIA

A group of pure AD can be delimited by postmortem findings, clinical investigations, laboratory data and brain imaging. Characteristics of this disorder are symptoms of parieto-temporal type and absence of general and confusional symptoms. There is no blood–brain barrier (BBB) damage and no substantial white-matter degeneration. Increased CSF–GM1 and decreased CSF-chromogranin A concentrations may be markers for the disease. Concerning the course of the disorder, there is insidious and early onset and a relatively slow progression of the disorder (Nyth, 1992). Concerning the severity and the globality, there is in the early stage a parieto-temporal localization and the disorder is disabling. The postmortem findings in this disorders are severe Alzheimer encephalopathy with numerous SPs and NFTs, as compared with nondemented individuals of the same age.

SDAT can be assumed to be a more heterogeneous group. The symptomatology consists of general cognitive and confusional symptoms, and there is often mild BBB damage along with white-matter degeneration. Low vitamin B12 levels may be present. The course of the disorder is late onset and a progression that is either slow or rapid (Nyth, 1992). The postmortem findings are presence of less pronounced Alzheimer encephalopathy, but frequently also white-matter degeneration or other age-related changes, such as Lewy bodies. SDAT can obviously be divided into further subgroups. White-matter lesions may delimit a white-matter dementia and deficiency of essential nutrients may delimit another form of dementia. It is obvious that, at high ages, the aging factor itself is such a risk factor for dementia that we also must assume a 'normal-involution dementia'. Possibly a senile dementia of Lewy-body type should also be delimited when postmortem histopathological findings in the form of Lewy bodies are present. Perhaps a group that can be called 'senile dementia of multifactorial type' should also be delimited. The aging factor together with vascular factors, nutritional factors and toxic factors may, when they are combined, cause dementia.

REFERENCES

Basun, H. (1993) Biological markers in Alzheimer's disease: diagnostic implications. Thesis. Stockholm Gerontology Research Center, Stockholm, Sweden.

Blennow, K., and Wallin, A. (1992) Clinical heterogeneity of probable Alzheimer's disease. *J. Geriatr. Psychiatry Neurol.*, **5**, 106–113.

Gottfries, J., Blennow, K., Wallin, A., and Gottfries, C. G. Classification of dementia using partial least square analysis. In preparation.

Heston, L. L., Mastri, A. R., Anderson, E., and White, J. (1981) Dementia of the Alzheimer type: clinical genetics natural history and associated conditions. *Arch. Gen. Psychiatry*, **38**, 1085–1090.

Höskuldsson, A. (1988) PLS regression methods. *J. Chemometrics*, **2**, 211–228.

Kraepelin, E. (1910) *Senile and Pre-senile Dementias.* Johann Ambrosius Barth, Leipzig, pp. 533–554, 593–632.

Landin, K., Blennow, K., Wallin, A., and Gottfries, C. G. (1993) Low blood pressure and blood glucose levels in Alzheimer's disease: Evidence for a hypometabolic disorder? *J. Intern. Med.*, **233**, 357–363.

Larsson, T., Sjögren, T., and Jacobson, G. (1963) Senile dementia. A clinical, sociomedical and genetic study. *Acta Psychiatr. Scand. Suppl.*, 167.

McKhann, G., Drachman, D., Folstein, M., Katzman, R., Price, D., and Stadlan, E. M. (1984) Clinical diagnosis of Alzheimer's disease: Report of the NINCDS-ADRDA Work Group under the auspices of Department of Health and Human Services Task Force on Alzheimer's Disease. *Neurology*, **34**, 939–944.

Nyth, A. L. (1992) Alzheimer's Disease—Aspects on Treatment and Course. Thesis. University of Göteborg, Sweden.

Regland, B., Gottfries, C. G., Oreland, L., and Svennerholm, L. (1988) Low B12 levels related to high activity of platelet MAO in patients with dementia disorders. A retrospective study. *Acta Psychiatr. Scand.*, **78**, 451–457.

Sjögren, T., Sjögren, H., and Lindgren, Å. (1952) Morbus Alzheimer and morbus Pick: a genetic, clinical and patho-anatomical study. *Acta Psychiatr. Neurol. Scand.* (suppl.), **82**, 66–115.

Sourander, P., and Sjögren, H. (1970) The concept of Alzheimer's disease and its clinical implications. In G. E. W. Wolstenholme and M. O'Connor (eds), *Alzheimer's Disease and Related Conditions.* Churchill, London, pp. 11–36.

2

Biochemical Aspects and CSF Markers in Alzheimer's Disease

K. Blennow, A. Wallin, and C. G. Gottfries

Department of Clinical Neuroscience, University of Göteborg, Mölndal, Sweden

ABSTRACT

A biochemical marker for Alzheimer's disease (AD) would be of great value, as it would improve the clinical diagnostic accuracy in scientific studies and increase our knowledge of the pathogenesis of the disorder. In this chapter, we present a clinical neurochemical approach in which several cerebrospinal fluid (CSF) biochemical markers are used together, to give a characteristic pattern. These CSF biochemical markers are divided into 'positive' markers, intended to reflect the underlying pathological processes in AD, and 'negative' markers, intended to reflect pathological processes that are unrelated to AD, such as cerebrovascular and ischemic lesions. Thus, negative markers may be used to exclude cases with mixed AD and vascular dementia. The list of potential positive CSF biochemical markers includes βA4 protein for amyloid deposition, hyperphosphorylated tau proteins for neurofibrillary tangles, neuron-specific enolase and ganglioside GM1 for neuronal degeneration, and chromogranin

Alzheimer's Disease: Clinical and Treatment Perspectives. Edited by N. R. Cutler, C. G. Gottfries and K. Siegfried.

A and synaptotagmin for synaptic degeneration. Potential negative CSF-biochemical markers are sulfatide for white-matter lesions (leukoaraiosis), and the CSF/serum albumin ratio for intracerebral small blood-vessel arteriolosclerosis.

INTRODUCTION

Alzheimer's disease (AD) is the most common cause of dementia, accounting for about 50% of all cases, and the third most common cause of death, after atherosclerosis (myocardial infarction and stroke) and cancer. In view of its high frequency and malignant natural course, AD can be said to be 'a major killer' (Katzman, 1986). The etiology of AD is unknown, and today there is no treatment than can cure or arrest the disease.

AD is characterized by progressive dementia with memory disturbances and instrumental symptoms (Sjögren *et al.*, 1952; Lishman, 1987). The neuropathological findings consist of degeneration of neurons and their synapses (Coleman and Flood, 1987; Davies *et al.*, 1987; Hamos *et al.*, 1989; Masliah *et al.*, 1989), and an increased number of senile plaques (SPs) and neurofibrillary tangles (NFTs) compared with that found in non-demented individuals of the same age (Tomlinson and Corsellis, 1984). Today, the clinical diagnosis of AD is made by way of exclusion (McKhann *et al.*, 1984), without any positive criteria. Therefore, biochemical markers for AD would be of great use in the attempts to improve the clinical diagnostic accuracy in scientific studies and treatment trials and to increase the knowledge of the pathogenesis of the disorder.

CONFOUNDING FACTORS FOR STUDIES ON CSF BIOCHEMICAL MARKERS FOR ALZHEIMER'S DISEASE

Clinical Diagnostic Accuracy

One of the major problems when studying biochemical markers for AD is that an incorrect clinical diagnosis may cause the potential of a biochemical marker to be overlooked. Today, the clinical diagnosis of AD is made by way of exclusion, without any positive items, using the NINCDS-ADRDA criteria for 'probable AD' (McKhann *et al.*, 1984). These criteria include: (1) the presence of progressive dementia, (2) no disturbance of consciousness at the time of diagnosis, (3) onset between ages 40 and 90, and (4) absence of systemic disorders or other brain diseases that alone could account for the dementia, e.g. manic-depressive disorder, Parkinson's disease, and multi-infarct dementia. No specifications are given how to deal with patients with cerebrovascular risk factors (e.g. hypertension) or brain-imaging findings of white-matter lesions (WMLs) (McKhann *et al.*, 1984).

It is clear that such vague exclusion criteria entail a risk of delimiting a heterogeneous group of patients. Several studies have also presented results suggesting that the current criteria for AD include at least two subgroups of patients. One subgroup (*AD type I*) is characterized by relatively early onset (mean 60 years of age), a characteristic cortical symptomatology of memory disturbances and instrumental ('parietal') symptoms, findings of marked degeneration of cortical neurons and synapses, and high numbers of cortical SPs and NFTs (for review see Blennow and Wallin, 1992). These characteristics match the classical description of Alzheimer's disease, and AD type I has therefore been suggested to constitute 'classical' or 'pure' AD. The other subgroup (*AD type II*) is characterized by relatively late onset (mean 72 years of age), a more generalized symptomatology, often concomitant vascular diseases, e.g. hypertension, and often findings of WMLs on CT or MRI (for review see Blennow and Wallin, 1992). These findings suggest that AD type II may have a 'mixed' pathogenesis, with an age-related lowered threshold for dementia and a combination of relatively mild Alzheimer-type and cerebrovascular changes.

When studying potential CSF biochemical markers for AD, we suggest that the results should also be evaluated using these subgroups. New research criteria to identify cases of 'pure' AD have been suggested (Wallin *et al.*, 1994).

Clinical Neurochemical Confounding Factors

Several drawbacks exist for analyses of biochemical markers in CSF. Unless these confounding factors are kept under control, the results may be incorrect, or the potential of a biochemical marker may be overlooked.

Some CSF proteins are present uniquely in the CSF (and not detectable in serum), e.g. tau protein (Vandermeeren *et al.*, 1993). However, if the protein is present both in serum and CSF, it must be determined to what extent there is a diffusion through the blood–brain barrier from serum to CSF. For example, using monoclonal antibodies against pancreatic thread protein (PTP), a protein was found that shares epitopes with PTP but has a higher MW than PTP (Ozturk *et al.*, 1989). This protein was called neural thread protein (NTP) and was found to be present in the CSF (de la Monte *et al.*, 1992). Analysing only CSF (and not serum), these authors found an increased CSF concentration of NTP in AD and suggested that CSF-NTP is a biochemical marker for AD (de la Monte *et al.*, 1992). However, NTP-immunoreactivity is also present in the serum, in a concentration about fifty times as high as that in the CSF (Blennow *et al.*, 1994a). After correction for the diffusion of NTP-immunoreactivity from serum to CSF through the blood–brain barrier, there was no difference in CSF-NTP between AD and controls (Blennow *et al.*, 1994a).

Other confounding factors for CSF analyses include influence of concentration gradients along the spinal cord (Blennow *et al.*, 1993a). These concentration gradients make it necessary to perform all CSF analyses on a standardized volume of CSF; it is always a European consensus to analyse the first 10–12 ml of the CSF.

POTENTIAL CSF BIOCHEMICAL MARKERS FOR ALZHEIMER'S DISEASE

Biochemical markers for AD may be divided into 'positive' and 'negative'. Positive markers reflect underlying pathological processes in AD, i.e. the degeneration of preferentially cortical neurons and synapses (Coleman and Flood, 1987; Masliah *et al.*, 1989) and the increased numbers of SPs and NFTs in AD patients as compared with non-demented individuals of the same age (Tomlinson and Corsellis, 1984). Negative markers identify pathological processes that are unrelated to AD, e.g. cerebrovascular and ischemic lesions, and may thus be used to identify cases of mixed AD and vascular dementia (VAD).

Positive Markers

Amyloid Deposition

The amyloid fibrils in the core of SPs consist of a protein of 39–43 amino acids called the *βA4 protein* (Joachim and Selkoe, 1992). βA4 protein is cleaved from a larger precursor protein, *amyloid precursor protein (APP)*, which has at least three isoforms containing the βA4 sequence (APP_{695}, APP_{751}, and APP_{770}) (Joachim and Selkoe, 1992). Soluble APP derivatives have been found to be present in the CSF. Studies on the capacity of CSF-APP as a diagnostic marker for AD have yielded contradictory results, ranging from a reduced to an increased 'total' APP concentration in the CSF, and with differences in the relations between APP isoforms (for review see Blennow *et al.*, 1993b). These discrepancies may have resulted from differences in analytical methods, in patient and control samples, or in CSF sample collection and handling, and call for further studies to clarify the potential of CSF-APP as a biochemical marker for amyloid deposition.

Until recently, βA4 protein had not been identified in the CSF, probably because it appears there only in low concentrations owing to its tendency to aggregate into insoluble polymers. However, βA4 protein has now been found to be generated continuously as a soluble protein during normal cellular metabolism (Haas *et al.*, 1992) and can be detected in the CSF and plasma by means of more sensitive assays (Seubert *et al.*, 1992). Thus, the measurement of βA4 protein in the CSF has a potential for reflecting cerebral amyloid deposition. So far, there have been no studies analysing βA4 protein in the CSF from large patient and control samples.

Neurofibrillary Tangles

NFTs consist of bundles of paired helical filaments (PHFs) that are twisted around each other and wound in a helical manner

(Joachim and Selkoe, 1992). Using the monoclonal antibody (MAb) 5–25 against PHFs, Metha and co-workers (1985) found high levels of 'paired helical filaments antigen' in the CSF from AD patients. However, further studies have revealed that the epitope recognized by MAb 5–25 is residues 64–76 of *ubiquitin* (Perry *et al.*, 1989), and that MAb 5–25 recognizes a variety of proteins conjugated to ubiquitin in CSF (Wang *et al.*, 1991). Ubiquitin (Ub) is a 76 amino acid (8.7 kDa) protein that is found in all eukaryotic cells. The best characterized function of Ub is its involvement in an ATP-dependent degradation of proteins in which Ub is covalently conjugated to the amino-group of lysine residues of target proteins, where it serves as a signal for degradation of the protein by proteases. However, Ub-conjugated proteins may also be stable and exist in the cell indefinitely. An example of this is the findings of ubiquinated NFTs in aging and in AD. A recent CSF study confirmed the finding of high ubiquitin immunoreactivity in AD (Wang *et al.*, 1991). Another CSF study found an increase in free ubiquitin in AD, but also in VAD (Blennow *et al.*, 1993c). Further studies are needed to characterize the ubiquitin-conjugated proteins recognized by MAb 5–25 in the CSF and to ascertain the cause of the up-regulation of the ubiquitin system in AD.

Hyperphosphorylated tau proteins are probably a major component of PHFs (Delacourte *et al.*, 1990; Lee *et al.*, 1991). Because of their phosphorylation, these tau proteins have a slightly higher MW (of 60–68 kDa) than normal tau (Lee *et al.*, 1991) and have been named *Tau 64* and *Tau 69* (Delacourte *et al.*, 1990). The Alz-50 MAb was produced against brain tissue homogenates from AD patients. In an initial study, Alz-50 was found to recognize a single protein with an MW of 68 kDa designated *A68* (Wolozin *et al.*, 1986). Later studies showed that A68 is one of three proteins (Lee *et al.*, 1991) or protein aggregates (Bisette *et al.*, 1991) with MWs of 60–68 kDa (Lee *et al.*, 1991), also called *Alzheimer's disease associated proteins (ADAP)* (Bisette *et al.*, 1991). A68/ADAP have been shown to be identical to the hyperphosphorylated tau proteins (Bisette *et al.*, 1991; Lee *et al.*, 1991) and to be greatly enriched in brains from patients with AD (Wolozin and Davies, 1987), especially in patients with early onset AD (Bisette *et al.*, 1991). Although hyperphosphorylated tau proteins have been shown to have low solubility (Delacourte *et al.*, 1990), they are present in the CSF in low concentrations (Wolozin and Davies, 1987) and have a potential as a diagnostic marker for AD.

Neuronal Degeneration

The gamma-gamma isoform of enolase, called *neuron-specific enolase (NSE)*, is a 78 kDa protein that, in the brain, is localized in the cytosol of neurons (Marangos, 1991). Increased CSF levels of NSE have been found in acute brain disorders, such as stroke and head trauma (Marangos, 1991). In chronic brain disorders, CSF-NSE may have a potential as a marker for neuronal degeneration. In a recent study, increased levels (187% of control values) of CSF-NSE were found in AD (Blennow *et al.*, 1994b). However, CSF-NSE was also elevated in VAD (177% of control values), and no difference in levels was found between AD type I and AD type II (Blennow *et al.*, 1994b), suggesting that CSF-NSE may be used as a non-disease-specific marker for neuronal degeneration.

Brain gangliosides are located in the neuronal membranes, but their subcellular location is insufficiently known. Some researchers argue that gangliosides are enriched in the synaptic region (Hansson *et al.*, 1977), whereas others claim that they are distributed over the entire neuronal membrane (Ledeen, 1985). We used a new method for the determination of the brain gangliosides GM1, GD1a, GD1b and GT1b in individual samples of CSF (Davidsson *et al.*, 1989). Markedly higher levels of CSF-*ganglioside GM1* were found in patients with 'pure' AD (AD type I) (273% of control values), whereas the CSF-GM1 levels in AD type II and VAD did not differ from those in controls (Blennow *et al.*, 1991a). These findings suggest that CSF-GM1 has a potential as a positive marker for 'pure' AD that is capable of identifying neuronal and synaptic degeneration. However, the sensitivity and specificity of CSF-GM1 as a diagnostic marker have to be further studied.

Synaptic Degeneration

Chromogranin A (CrA) is a soluble 70–75 kDa protein that, in the brain, is localized in the large dense-core vesicles of the synapses, and is absent in the small synaptic vesicles (Winkler *et al.*, 1986). While cortical brain tissue homogenates from AD patients show a decrease in markers for small synaptic vesicles, such as synaptophysin, an increase in CrA has been found (Lassman *et al.*, 1992). It has also been shown that CrA accumulates in the dystrophic neurites in SPs in AD (Munoz, 1991; Lassman *et al.*, 1992). Thus, CSF-CrA may have a potential as a marker for synaptic pathology. When we determined CrA in CSF using a sandwich ELISA method, CSF-CrA was reduced in AD type I (68% of control values), while the levels of CSF-CrA in AD type II and in VAD were normal (Blennow *et al.*, unpublished data). The lower CSF concentration of CrA in AD type I may reflect synaptic degeneration in this subgroup of AD, or alternatively, a deposition of CrA in the dystrophic neurites in SPs.

Synaptotagmin is a 65 kDa protein that is localized in the membrane of the small synaptic vesicles in the brain (for review see Jessell and Kandel, 1993). Cortical brain tissue homogenates from AD patients show a decrease in markers for small synaptic vesicles, such as synaptophysin and synaptotagmin (Lassman *et al.*, 1992), probably reflecting a severe loss of cortical synapses in AD. Preliminary data from our department show that synaptotagmin is present in the CSF (Davidsson *et al.*, unpublished data). Further studies of the potential of CSF synaptotagmin as a biochemical marker for the synaptic degeneration in AD are in progress.

Negative CSF Markers

White-matter Lesions

In recent years, after the introduction of high-resolution CT, and later MRI, WMLs, often called leukoaraiosis, have been a frequent finding in patients fulfilling the criteria for probable AD, preferentially those with late onset AD (AD type II) (Wallin *et al.*, 1989; Blennow *et al.*, 1991b; Scheltens *et al.*, 1992). This periventricular white-matter demyelination is associated with aging and dementia. Many studies have also shown a relation between WMLs and hypertension, suggesting a cerebrovascular origin of

WMLs (for review see Blennow and Wallin, 1992). Thus, although their pathogenesis is insufficiently known, WMLs are probably often of vascular origin, and may be used as a 'negative' marker for AD. To find a possible marker for demyelination, and thereby also WMLs, we developed an assay for determining the CSF content of *sulfatide,* the major acidic glycosphingolipid in the myelin sheaths of the nerve cells (Fredman *et al.*, 1992). High CSF concentrations of sulfatide were found in VAD, 212% of control values; a slight (130% of control values), but statistically not significant, increase was found in AD type II, while the concentration was normal in AD type I (Fredman *et al.*, 1992). These findings suggest that CSF-sulfatide has a potential as a negative biochemical marker for 'pure AD' (AD type I).

Small Blood-vessel Arteriosclerosis

In neuropathological studies, a small blood-vessel arteriolosclerosis is often found in patients with WMLs (for review see Blennow and Wallin, 1992). The blood–brain barrier (BBB) is situated in the small vessels of the brain. Thus, the *CSF/S albumin ratio,* a measure of the BBB function, may serve as a measure of cerebral small-vessel damage. In a CSF study on BBB function in dementia disorders, the CSF/S albumin ratio was normal in AD type I, but elevated in AD type II and VAD (Blennow *et al.*, 1990, 1991b). The elevation was probably related to damage to the small intracerebral blood vessels in these disorders and was found preferentially in patients with WMLs (Blennow *et al.*, 1990, 1991b). These findings suggest that examinations of the BBB function is important to identify 'pure' AD (AD type I).

CONCLUSIONS

Since the neuropathological findings in AD are not specific—they also occur in other disorders and in normal aging (Wisniewski *et al.*, 1979)—there is little hope of ever finding a single biochemical marker specific for AD. However, this

Table 1 *Potential cerebrospinal fluid biochemical markers for pure Alzheimer's disease*

	'Positive'	'Negative'
Amyloid deposition	βA4 protein Amyloid precursor protein (APP)	
Neurofibrillary tangles	Tau protein Hyperphosphorylated tau protein (Tau 64/69; A68/ADAP)	
Neuronal degeneration	Gangliosides Neuron specific enolase	
Synaptic degeneration		
Large dense-core vesicles	Chromogranin A	
Small synaptic vesicles	Synaptotagmin	
White-matter lesions		Sulfatide
Blood–brain dysfunction		CSF/S albumin ratio

ADAP = Alzheimer's disease associated proteins.

drawback can be overcome if several CSF-markers, each reflecting a pathological process, are used together to give a pattern characteristic of AD (Table 1).

Thus, we suggest that CSF biochemical markers for AD may include a characteristic pattern of 'positive' CSF-biochemical markers (reflecting processes related to AD, such as neuronal and synaptic degeneration, amyloid deposition and NFTs), and CSF concentrations within the normal range for 'negative' biochemical markers (reflecting processes not related to AD, such as WMLs and BBB damage).

REFERENCES

Bisette, G., Smith, W. H., Dole, K. C., *et al.* (1991) Alterations in Alzheimer's disease-associated protein in Alzheimer's disease frontal and temporal cortex. *Arch. Gen. Psychiatry*, **48**, 1009–1012.

Blennow, K., and Wallin, A. (1992) Clinical heterogeneity of probable Alzheimer's disease. *J. Geriatr. Psychiatry Neurol.*, **5**, 106–113.

Blennow, K., Wallin, A., Fredman, P., *et al.* (1990) Blood–brain barrier disturbance in patients with Alzheimer's disease is related to vascular factors. *Acta Neurol. Scand.*, **81**, 323–326.

Blennow, K., Davidsson, P., Wallin, A., *et al.* (1991a) Gangliosides in cerebrospinal fluid in probable Alzheimer's disease. *Arch. Neurol.*, **48**, 1032–1035.

Blennow, K., Wallin, A., Uhlemann, C., *et al.* (1991b) White-matter lesions on CT in Alzheimer patients: relation to clinical symptomatology and vascular factors. *Acta Neurol. Scand.*, **83**, 187–193.

Blennow, K., Wallin, A., Gottfries, C. G., Månsson, J. E., and Svennerholm, L. (1993a) Concentration gradients for monoamine metabolites in lumbar cerebrospinal fluid. *J. Neural Transm.*, **5**, 5–15.

Blennow, K., Wallin, A., and Gottfries, C. G. (1993b) Cerebrospinal fluid biochemical markers for Alzheimer's disease. In E. C. Wolters and P. Scheltens (eds), *Alzheimer's Disease: Back to the Future.* ICG Printing, Dordrecht, pp. 29–38.

Blennow, K., Davidsson, P., Wallin, A., Gottfries, C. G. and Svennerholm, L. (1993c) Ubiquitin in cerebrospinal fluid in 'probable Alzheimer's disease'. *Psychogeriatrics Int.*, **6**, 13–22.

Blennow, K., Chong, J. K., and Wallin, A. (1994a) 'Neural thread protein' in cerebrospinal fluid comes from serum by passage over the blood–brain barrier. Submitted.

Blennow, K., Wallin, A., and Ekman, R. (1994b) Neuron-specific enolase in cerebrospinal fluid: a biochemical marker for neuronal degeneration in dementia disorders? Submitted.

Coleman, P. D., and Flood, D. G. (1987) Neuron numbers and dendrite extent in normal aging and Alzheimer's disease. *Neurobiol. Aging*, **8**, 521–545.

Davidsson, P., Fredman, P., and Svennerholm, L. (1989) Gangliosides and sulfatide in human cerebrospinal fluid: quantitation with immunoaffinity techniques. *J. Chromatogr.*, **496**, 279–289.

Davies, C. A., Mann, D. M. A., Sumpter, P. Q., and Yates, P. O. (1987) A quantitative morphometric analysis of the neuronal and synaptic content of the frontal and temporal cortex in patients with Alzheimer's disease. *J. Neurol. Sci.*, **78**, 151–164.

Delacourte, A., Flament, S., Dibe, E. M., *et al.* (1990) Pathological proteins Tau 64 and 69 are specifically expressed in the somatodendritic domain of the degenerating cortical neurons during Alzheimer's disease. *Acta Neuropathol.*, **80**, 111–117.

De la Monte, S., Growdon, J. H., Volicer, L., *et al.* (1992) Increased levels of neuronal thread protein in cerebrospinal fluid of patients with probable Alzheimer's disease. *Neurobiol. Aging*, **13**, 102.

Fredman, P., Wallin, A., Blennow, K., *et al.* (1992) Sulfatide as a biochemical marker in cerebrospinal fluid of patients with vascular dementia. *Acta Neurol. Scand.*, **85**, 103–106.

Haass, C., Schlossmacher, M. G., Hung, A. Y., *et al.* (1992) Amyloid β-peptide is produced by cultured cells during normal metabolism. *Nature*, **359**, 322–325.

Hamos, J. E., DeGennaro, L. J., and Drachman, D. A. (1989) Synaptic loss in Alzheimer's disease and other dementias. *Neurology*, **39**, 355–361.

Hansson, H. A., Holmgren, J., and Svennerholm, L. (1977) Ultrastructural localization of cell membrane GM1 ganglioside by cholera toxin. *Proc. Natl Acad. Sci. USA*, **74**, 3782–3786.

Jessel, T. M. and Kandel, E. R. (1993) Synaptic transmission: a bidirectional and self-modifiable form of cell–cell communication. *Cell*, **10** (Suppl. 1), 1–30.

Joachim, C. L., and Selkoe, D. J. (1992) The seminal role of β-amyloid in the pathogenesis of Alzheimer's disease. *Alz. Dis. Assoc. Disord.*, **6**, 7–34.

Katzman, R. (1986) Alzheimer's disease. *N. Engl. J. Med.*, **314**, 964–973.

Lassmann, H., Weiler, R., Fischer, P., *et al.* (1992) Synaptic pathology in Alzheimer's disease: immunological data for markers for synaptic and large dense-core vesicles. *Neuroscience*, **46**, 1–8.

Ledeen, R. (1985) Gangliosides of the neuron. *Trends Neurosci.*, **8**, 169–175.

Lee, V. M. Y., Balin, B. J., Otvos, L., *et al.* (1991) A68: a major subunit of paired helical filaments and derivatized forms of normal tau. *Science*, **251**, 675–679.

Lishman, W. A. (1987) *Organic Psychiatry, the Psychological Consequences of Cerebral Disorder*. 2nd edn. Year Book Medical Publishers, Chicago.

Marangos, P. J. (1991) Neuron specific enolase as a clinical tool in neurologic and endocrine disease. In M. Gratzl and K. Langley (eds), *Markers for Neural and Endocrine Cells*. VCH, Weinheim, pp. 181–189.

Masliah, E., Terry, R. D., DeTeresa, R. M., *et al.* (1989) Immunohistochemical quantification of the synapse-related protein synaptophysin in Alzheimer's disease. *Neurosci Lett.*, **103**, 234–239.

McKhann, G., Drachman, D., Folstein, M., *et al.* (1984) Clinical diagnosis of Alzheimer's disease: report of the NINCDS-ADRDA Work Group under the auspices of department of health and human services task force on Alzheimer's disease. *Neurology*, **34**, 939–944.

Metha, P. H., Thal, L., Wisniewski, H. M., *et al.* (1985) Paired helical filaments antigen in CSF. (letter). *Lancet*, **ii**, 35.

Munoz, D. G. (1991) Chromogranin A-like immunoreactive neurites are major constituents of senile plaques. *Lab. Invest*, **64**, 826–832.

Ozturk, M., de la Monte, S., Gross, J., *et al.* (1989) Elevated levels of an exocrine pancreatic secretory protein in Alzheimer disease brain. *Proc. Natl Acad. Sci. USA*, **86**, 419–423.

Perry, G., Mulvihill, P., Fried, V. A., *et al.* (1989) Immunochemical properties of ubiquitin conjugates in the paired helical filaments of Alzheimer disease. *J. Neurochem.*, **52**, 1523–1528.

Scheltens, P., Barkhof, F., Valk, J., *et al.* (1992) White matter lesions on magnetic resonance imaging in Alzheimer's disease: evidence for heterogeneity. *Brain*, **115**, 735–748.

Seubert, P., Vigo-Pelfrey, C., Esch, F., *et al.* (1992) Isolation and quantification of soluble Alzheimer's β-peptide from biological fluids. *Nature*, **359**, 325–327.

Sjögren, T., Sjögren, H., and Lindgren, Å. (1952) Morbus Alzheimer and morbus Pick: A genetic, clinical and patho-anatomical study. *Acta Psychiatr. Neurol. Scand.* (Suppl. 82), 66–115.

Tomlinson, B. E., and Corsellis, J. A. N. (1984) Ageing and the dementias. In J. Hume Adams, J. A. N. Corsellis, and L. W. Duchen (eds), *Greenfield's Neuropathology*. Edward Arnold, London, pp. 951–1025.

Vandermeeren, M., Mercken, M., Vanmechelen, E., Six, J., Van de Voorde, A., Martin, J. J. and Cras, P. (1993) Detection of proteins in normal and Alzheimer's disease cerebrospinal fluid with a sensitive sandwich enzyme-linked immunosorbent assay. *J. Neurochem.*, **61**, 1828–1834.

Wallin, A., Blennow, K., Uhlemann, C., *et al.* (1989) White matter low attenuation on computed tomography in Alzheimer's disease and vascular dementia—diagnostic and pathogenetic aspects. *Acta Neurol. Scand.*, **80**, 518–523.

Wallin, A., Blennow, K., and Scheltens, P. (1994) Research criteria for clinical diagnosis of 'pure' Alzheimer's disease. *Drugs of Today*, **30**, 265–273.

Wang, G. P., Iqbal, K., Bucht, G., *et al.* (1991) Alzheimer's disease: paired helical filament immunoreactivity in cerebrospinal fluid. *Acta Neuropathol.*, **82**, 6–12.

Winkler, H., Apps, D. K., and Fischer-Colbrie, R. (1986) The molecular function of adrenal chromaffin granules: established facts and unresolved topics. *Neuroscience*, **18**, 261–290.

Wisniewski, K., Jervis, G. A., Moretz, R. C., *et al.* (1979) Alzheimer neurofibrillary tangles in diseases other than senile and presenile dementia. *Ann. Neurol.*, **5**, 288–294.

Wolozin, B., and Davies, P. (1987) Alzheimer-related neuronal protein A68: specificity and distribution. *Ann. Neurol.*, **22**, 521–526.

Wolozin, B. L., Pruchnicki, A., Dickson, D. W., *et al.* (1986) A neuronal antigen in the brains of Alzheimer patients. *Science*, **232**, 648–650.

3
Brain Imaging and Alzheimer's Disease

Ph. Scheltens

Department of Neurology, Vrije Universiteit, Amsterdam, The Netherlands

ABSTRACT

In this chapter the contribution of CT and MRI to the diagnosis of Alzheimer's disease (AD) is reviewed. Special attention is given to the assessment of general brain atrophy and temporal lobe atrophy. The specific contribution of MRI to the differential diagnosis of AD is addressed, as well as the combination of MRI and functional studies.

It is concluded that CT may be used for the exclusion of other causes of dementia. Finding cortical or subcortical atrophy on CT or MRI itself does not indicate AD, unless an increase in CSF volume over a period of one year is documented. Reviewing the available data on hippocampal atrophy on CT/MRI, it seems more than speculative that it may provide a useful early marker. CT and MRI based measurements of hippocampal atrophy have been shown to provide useful diagnostic information for separating patients with probable AD from normal elderly individuals.

The use of a standardized imaging protocol, including some assessment of hippocampal atrophy, can be considered a cost-

Alzheimer's Disease: Clinical and Treatment Perspectives. Edited by N. R. Cutler, C. G. Gottfries and K. Siegfried.

effective approach. In the evaluation of patients with dementia, they must undergo a cross-sectional imaging study to exclude other (treatable) causes of dementia. For scientific studies, volumetric measurements will be mandatory, because of the incorporation of adjustment for age and intracranial volume. This is best done on MRI. However, in clinical practice, simple visual inspection, using either CT or MRI, may provide the clinician with ample diagnostic information with respect to the presence of AD, although the value as a specific diagnostic marker for AD has to be proven in a sample representative of the general population.

Combining either assessment of hippocampal atrophy with cerebral blood flow measurements on SPECT does not seem to be warranted both from a clinical and economical point of view.

INTRODUCTION

The clinical diagnosis of Alzheimer's disease (AD) has been greatly facilitated by the introduction of specific diagnostic research criteria for AD, such as the NINCDS-ADRDA criteria (McKhann *et al.*, 1984) and the DSM-III R (American Psychiatric Association, 1987). This marked a shift from a purely exclusionary approach towards a diagnostic strategy in which specific clinical features are used to identify AD. However, the diagnosis still depends on the exclusion of other dementing illnesses that may mimic the clinical findings of AD. In most studies (Kukull *et al.*, 1990; Lopez *et al.*, 1990) the aforementioned criteria have a modest inter-observer agreement (55–75%) and clinical–pathological agreement ranges from 65 to 100% (Tierney *et al.*, 1988; Jellinger, 1990). Therefore, an urgent need has arisen for an objective diagnostic marker for the clinical diagnosis of AD. This would not only improve clinical diagnostic accuracy and would enable clinical research in other forms of dementia, but would also benefit future therapeutic trials in AD (Scheltens *et al.*, 1992b). Since there is no biological marker obtainable in blood or cerebrospinal fluid (CSF) and brain biopsy for diagnosing AD in clinical practice is far from feasible, neuro-imaging modalities have served this purpose for a great many years.

Computed tomography (CT) of the brain has been studied extensively during the past decade and has proven not to be very specific for AD. Since the beginning of the 1980s magnetic resonance imaging (MRI), as a new morphologic and safe imaging modality, has been available for routine practice and has become the new gold standard for imaging the central nervous system (Valk and van der Knaap, 1989). In comparison to CT it has several advantages, like absence of X-rays and beam-hardening artifacts. Paired with a higher contrast resolution (gray/white matter and brain/CSF) and the possibility of multiplanar imaging without the patient having to change position makes MRI highly suitable to study the aging brain in greater detail (Drayer, 1988), and to obtain information that was previously unrecognized in vivo (Press *et al.*, 1989).

In the following I will review the contribution of CT and MRI to the diagnosis of AD. I will focus on the assessment of general brain atrophy and temporal lobe atrophy in particular. The role of white matter changes will not be dealt with in this chapter. The specific contribution of MRI to the differential diagnosis of AD will be addressed, as well as the combination of MRI and functional studies.

GENERAL CEREBRAL ATROPHY

Cross-sectional Studies of General Brain Atrophy

During nearly two decades a vast number of studies has evaluated the diagnostic value of the assessment of general brain atrophy in AD by means of several neuroimaging techniques. Assessment of brain atrophy in the diagnosis of AD in vivo is based on neuropathological observations in AD. Loss of cortical and subcortical neurons accompanied by axonal dropout in the white matter, together with the formation of senile plaques and neurofibrillary tangles, result in reduced brain weight, cortical atrophy and ventricular enlargement in AD patients. However, since these changes also occur in normal aging, to a certain extent, there is a considerable overlap (Tomlinson *et al.*, 1968). Most studies have evaluated the value of CT/MRI to detect these changes in order to differentiate AD from normal aging.

The interpretation of those studies can be divided according to their methodology into (a) qualitative assessment, (b) linear measurements, (c) planimetric measurements and (d) volumetric measurements.

Qualitative Assessment

Qualitative (subjective) rating has been used to assess ventricular size and cortical atrophy. Studies on normal aging revealed significant correlations with age (Jacoby *et al.*, 1980a; Laffey *et al.*, 1984; Leys *et al.*, 1989) and a positive correlation between cortical atrophy and ventricular enlargement in most studies (Leys *et al.*, 1989; Baxter and Sorenson, 1981; Le May *et al.*, 1986). Due to considerable overlap with normal aging, subjective rating has little value for the diagnosis of AD. Moreover, this kind of assessment is highly dependent upon the raters' experience and has a low inter-observer reliability (De Carli *et al.*, 1990).

Linear Measurements

Linear measurements of the ventricular system and sulcal width are usually performed by computing the ratio of the distance between two points of interest and the width between the inner tables of the skull. In AD patients, ventricular widths, especially of the 3rd and lateral ventricles, differed significantly from age matched controls in most studies (Leys *et al.*, 1989; Jacoby *et al.*, 1980b; Brinkman *et al.*, 1981; Albert *et al.*, 1984b). Linear measurements of the temporal horns proved to be the most specific, although less sensitive (Le May *et al.*, 1986; Kido *et al.*, 1989). The method is limited, mainly because of inaccuracies in measuring the edges between ventricles and brain (Jacoby *et al.*, 1980b) and also because of a low inter-observer reliability. Although MRI lacks some of these disadvantages, linear measurements on MRI have not been performed frequently. Schmidt (1992) reported that ventricular enlargement on MRI was correlated with dementia severity in AD and that widening of the 3rd ventricle was the most sensitive predictor of AD.

Planimetric Measurements

Planimetry involves measurements of the area of regions of interest, either by manual tracing or computer assistance. This method enables measurements of ventricular area, the best estimate being the ventricular brain ratio (VBR) which is the ratio of the ventricular surface and brain area at a certain level (Zatz *et al.*, 1982; Zatz and Jernigan, 1983). Planimetry offers a better estimate of ventricular size than linear measurements, and is a more sensitive and specific method for the differentiation of AD patients from age-matched controls. However, it suffers from limitations in determining the size of the ventricular system based on a single level and is influenced by variation in normal anatomy and positioning of the head within the scanner (Penn *et al.*, 1978). The limitations of planimetric measurement can be overcome in part by obtaining volumetric measurements.

Volumetric Measurements

Two major techniques exist to determine the volumes of various cerebrospinal fluid (CSF) spaces. One method involves outlining a region of interest (ROI) with summation of cross-sectional areas of the ROI on each CT/MRI slice on which it appears, taking into account the slice thickness and the interslice distance (Turkheimer *et al.*, 1984). Another method involves obtaining Hounsfield unit (HU) values on CT, representative of typical CSF and brain regions, to determine an appropriate HU threshold value that optimally separates brain from CSF pixels and then counting the number of pixels above and below this particular HU value. Both methods have been found to be reliable to examine CSF spaces. There is a highly significant linear correlation between VBR and CSF volumes, suggesting that VBR is also a reliable method to estimate CSF volumes (Penn *et al.*, 1978). CSF volume increases with age (Takeda and Matsuzawa, 1985a), in a nonlinear fashion: the size of the CSF space increases exponentially after the age of 40 years in men and after the age of 50 years in women (Takeda and Matsuzawa, 1985b).

In AD, mean volumes of CSF spaces even in mildly impaired patients are approximately two times greater than in controls

(Gado *et al.*, 1982; Albert *et al.*, 1984a). The same was found recently by Sullivan *et al.* (1993) who also showed that early onset AD patients were quantitatively more abnormal than and showed a different pattern of abnormality from late onset patients. Volumetric methods prove to be the most sensitive and specific with values approaching an accuracy of 90% in diagnosing AD (De Carli *et al.*, 1990).

With respect to MRI two developments in this field have to be mentioned. Computerized segmentation techniques on MRI can produce accurate volumetric measurements of CSF and brain volumes. In a study of 16 AD patients and 16 controls Tanna *et al.* (1991) found that AD patients had 49% more total CSF, 37% more extraventricular and 99% more ventricular volume, and 7% less brain volume than controls. This method has a very high interrater reliability. Another method consists of the measurement of cerebral gray matter volume using dual sequence MRI, with compensation for partial volume averaging. In a study of 14 AD patients and an equal number of controls, Rusinek *et al.* (1991) showed that AD patients had 45% less gray matter volume than controls, with the most significant reduction located at the temporal lobes. No differences in white matter content were noted.

Recently, Sandor *et al.* (1992) compared the value of volumetric CT and MRI measurements of nine comparable areas in differentiating AD patients from controls. Although volumetric estimations of several ROIs on both imaging modalities significantly differed between the two groups, a discriminant function analysis selected only the first two variables from the MRI data set, which significantly differentiated 95% of the AD patients from controls. These two ROIs were the area of the lateral ventricle and the area of the Sylvian fissure. This study indicates that volumetric MRI measurements have a smaller measurement error than CT measurements.

Longitudinal Studies of General Cerebral Atrophy

Longitudinal studies have been performed using linear, planimetric and volumetric measurements of ventricular size (Gado *et al.*, 1982; Luxenberg *et al.*, 1987; Brinkman and Largen,

1984; De Leon *et al.*, 1989a; Leys *et al.*, 1990). It has been shown that the changes in lateral ventricular volume are the most predictive of AD, but not in an early stage (De Carli *et al.*, 1992). The rate of ventricular enlargement, with each method, is significantly higher in AD patients than in normal aging and correlates strongly with the decline of cognitive functions. When volumetric or planimetric measures are incorporated into longitudinal analysis it may dramatically increase the sensitivity and the specificity for the clinical diagnosis of AD towards 100%.

TEMPORAL LOBE ATROPHY

The hippocampus and adjacent structures situated in the medial temporal lobe are crucial to memory. Their bilateral destruction invariably leads to memory loss (Scoville and Milner, 1957; Zola-Morgan *et al.*, 1986; Damasio *et al.*, 1985). Memory impairment is an early, prominent manifestation of AD, and the hippocampal formation and parahippocampal gyrus are among the brain areas most consistently and heavily implicated in its pathology, even in an early stage (Braak *et al.*, 1993). Ball *et al.* (1985) have stated that AD is mainly a 'hippocampal dementia' by demonstrating nerve cell loss and gliosis in both hippocampi of AD patients while other brain regions were unaffected. Other studies referring to the pathology of AD have also incriminated the temporal basal gray-matter structures, including the hippocampus, as the earliest and most severely involved brain areas in AD (Tierney *et al.*, 1988). It therefore seems logical that neuroimaging studies have focused on these areas, to detect structural changes at an early stage. CT of the temporal lobes, however, is hampered by bone hardening artifact and limited view angle; it visualizes enlargement of the temporal horns and widening of the hippocampal fissures as indirect changes due to atrophy of the hippocampal complex. With MRI, better visualization of the medial temporal lobes, including the hippocampus, became available. This is mainly due to absence of bone hardening artifacts, and the possibility of imaging in a plane perpendicular to the long axis of the hippocampus, thus reducing volume averaging. This technique permits direct visualization of the hippocampal formation in substantial cytoarchitectonic detail (Press *et al.*, 1989).

CT Studies

CT studies in which cerebrospinal fluid (CSF) spaces in the anterior temporal region were subjectively assessed have claimed a modest accuracy in separating AD patients from elderly controls (LeMay *et al.*, 1986; Kido *et al.*, 1989; George *et al.*, 1990; Sandor *et al.*, 1988). In the study by LeMay *et al.* (1986) CT scans of 24 AD patients and 22 controls were compared. Perceptual ratings of atrophy of the temporal lobe regions produced an average accuracy of 87%. An accuracy of 94% was found by Sandor *et al.* (1988) using a similar CT technique and assessments. However, this excellent result was achieved only when subjects younger than 65 years were analysed separately from those aged 65 years and older. In another study (Kido *et al.*, 1989), temporal lobe atrophy was assessed by evaluating the temporal horns and Sylvian cisterns. Temporal horn measurements greater than 3 mm occurred only in AD patients, while measurements less than or equal to this occurred in both AD patients and controls. Subjective evaluation of the Sylvian cistern indicated that 24/29 controls had normal appearing cisterns while only 5/39 AD patients had similar findings. In contrast with the temporal horns, Sylvian cisterns proved to be more sensitive but less specific as discriminators between AD patients and controls. In 1993 Willmer *et al.* confirmed that specific measurements of the temporal lobes and horns yielded 92% correct classification of AD patients versus normal controls.

The first CT studies focusing only on the hippocampus (George *et al.*, 1990; De Leon *et al.*, 1989b) reported a significant widening of the hippocampal fissure, as indicator of hippocampal atrophy in AD patients, using a scanning angle 10–20° negative to the orbito-meatal line and parallel to the long axis of the hippocampus (Figure 1). In a cohort of 175 patients and controls, De Leon *et al.* (1989b) found that the sensitivity for AD ranged from 75 to 95%, increasing with the age of the subjects studied. Specificity, however, dropped markedly after the age of 60 years (from 100% before 60 years to 25% between 70 and 79 years). In a longitudinal follow-up study a group of non-demented elderly (n=28) and a group with questionable dementia (n=20) were followed for three years. Over the interval, 11 of 20 of the questionable group and 1 of 28 of the controls deteriorated to receive the clinical diagnosis of AD. Baseline hippocampal ratings ≥ 2, according to their scoring system, were present in 91% of the decliners and absent in 81% of the non-decliners (De Leon *et al.*, 1992).

In a study which included 51 AD patients and 18 controls, Jobst *et al.* (1992a) measured the average thickness of the medial

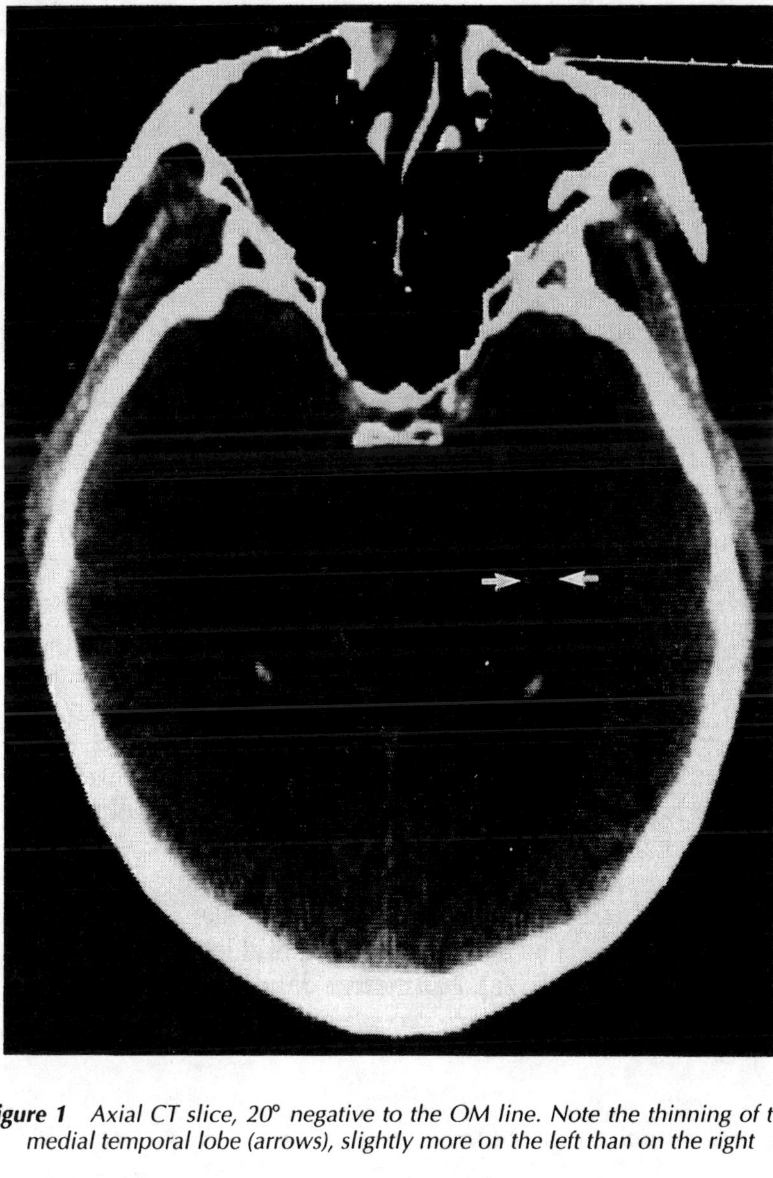

Figure 1 *Axial CT slice, 20° negative to the OM line. Note the thinning of the medial temporal lobe (arrows), slightly more on the left than on the right*

temporal lobe (hippocampal formation and gyrus) on axial CT slices made with the same negative angle protocol. They found that, using a medial temporal lobe thickness of 11.5 mm as cut-off value for hippocampal atrophy, 49/51 AD patients fell below this value, indicating hippocampal atrophy. Only 5/18 of the controls had a value below this cut-off value. Interestingly, 6/10 patients with other types of 'dementia' (vascular dementia, PSP, major depression) also had atrophy of the medial temporal lobe according to this criterion. Neuropathological examination revealed a diagnosis of AD in 10 patients, all of whom had shown CT evidence of hippocampal atrophy, including one patient with vascular dementia from the group with 'other types of dementia'. Very recently, the same authors confirmed their results in a larger study, in which they had data on 44 autopsy confirmed AD cases and 10 autopsy confirmed non-AD cases (Jobst *et al.*, 1992b). This study led to sheer optimism; however, it was firmly criticized by De Leon *et al.* (1993) in stating that the procedure should be applied to less impaired patients first before it could serve as a real diagnostic test for AD. Similar criticisms were made by Philbot and Burns (1993).

MRI Studies

MRI holds more promising options in detecting hippocampal atrophy. Using high resolution MRI in the coronal plane, T1-weighted images reveal the hippocampal formation in great detail. With advanced post-processing techniques, either by hand tracing or region growing, volumetric measurements of this structure are within reach. This technique has also been used to measure hippocampal volume of patients being evaluated for surgery for medically intractable epilepsy and an excellent correspondence has been found between the atrophic hippocampus, as assessed by MRI, and the site of the active epileptogenic focus as detected by temporal lobe EEGs and lobectomy (Jack *et al.*, 1992a). Normative data for the hippocampus and the temporal lobe were recently published by Bhatia *et al.* (1993).

The first study in AD patients was published in 1988, but remained uncited for a long time (Seab *et al.*, 1988). Volumetric measurements of the hippocampus in ten AD patients and seven control subjects revealed a 40% reduction in the AD group, without any overlap with controls. In addition, the authors showed that this reduction in hippocampal volume did not parallel, and probably preceded, overall brain atrophy. In a small study of three amnesic patients and four controls, Press *et al.* (1989) confirmed that MRI is able to produce highly detailed images of the hippocampus. The abnormalities that they could identify did contribute subsantially to the memory disturbances in their patients. Kesslak *et al.* (1991) studied eight AD patients and seven age-matched controls using coronal inversion recovery T1-weighted MR images. Volumetric measurements of the hippocampus and parahippocampal gyrus yielded values significantly lower in AD patients than in controls. They were able to separate the two groups completely. Moreover, they found good correlations between the observed atrophy and the severity of dementia measured by the mini mental state examination (Folstein *et al.*, 1975). Similar results were published recently by Killiany *et al.* (1993). Ikeda *et al.* (1994) showed that hippocampal and parahippocampal atrophy probably occur in early AD, since they found similar values both in possible and probable AD.

The excellent results of previously mentioned studies were probably biased because only very small groups were studied. This was illustrated by another study related to this topic (Jack *et al.*, 1992b) in which 20 AD patients and 22 controls were involved. This study convincingly showed that volumetric measurements of the hippocampus were sensitive in separating the two groups, but with a substantial overlap. Similar results were recently published by Pearlson *et al.* (1992). A recent observation by Cuenod *et al.* (1993) drew attention to atrophy of the amygdala, which may occur earlier than hippocampal atrophy.

A different approach was applied by Scheltens *et al.* (1992a) and Erkinjuntti *et al.* (1993). In a study involving 21 AD patients and an equal number of age-matched controls, the former authors reported significant differences in visually assessed hippocampal atrophy. They found a sensitivity of 81% and a specificity of 67%. In addition, they reported that linear measures of the medial temporal lobe correlated well with visual assessment, thus validating the clinical utility of their rating scale. Neuropsychological assessments of recent memory, in contrast to mental speed and attention, correlated highly with visually rated hippocampal atrophy, again stressing the unique involvement of this structure in AD patients together with its close relations to symptoms. The latter authors concluded that the presence of rated atrophy in selected temporal structures makes the diagnosis of AD more likely but the absence does not rule out the possibility of early AD.

An example of hippocampal atrophy on MRI is given in Figure 2.

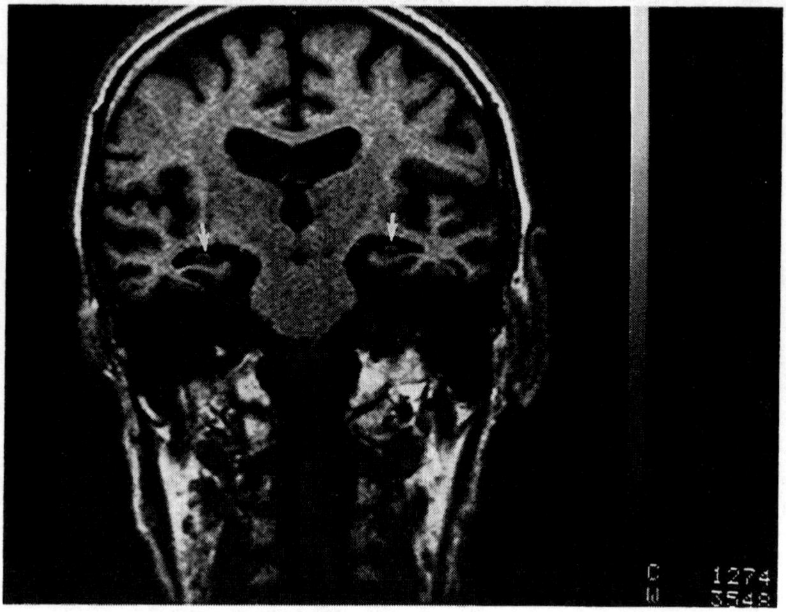

Figure 2 *T1-weighted (IR sequence) MR image in the coronal plane showing hippocampal atrophy (arrows)*

Some general remarks about the aforementioned studies have to be made. In most studies the clinical diagnosis of probable AD, according to current research criteria (McKhann *et al.*, 1984), was used as the 'gold standard'. Since the accuracy of these criteria in predicting the pathological diagnosis of AD is far from perfect, some questions can be raised about the validity of using these criteria against which to assess the value of a new diagnostic tool. Furthermore, it is not yet known if hippocampal atrophy on MRI occurs only in AD patients. Hippocampal abnormalities have also been reported in schizophrenics, amnesic patients and in subjects following severe hypoxia (Altshuler *et al.*, 1990). Moreover, healthy elderly displaying recent memory impairment also show evidence of hippocampal atrophy (Golomb *et al.*, 1993). Although this may imply subclinical AD, as was suggested by Ikeda *et al.* (1994), it may also be a normal phenomenon.

DIFFERENTIAL DIAGNOSIS

AD accounts for more than 60% of all dementias, while 40% may be caused by approximately 70 disorders. By stringent application of current research criteria to diagnose AD clinically, the majority of the other disorders will be ruled out, a process in which CT has been proven the most helpful (Engel and Gelber, 1992). However, in cases fulfilling NINCDS criteria (McKhann *et al.*, 1984) diagnostic uncertainty remains in about 10–20% (Jellinger, 1990; Lopez *et al.*, 1990; Tierney *et al.*, 1988). Apart from ruling out other diseases CT/MRI should also give important diagnostic information in those cases that fulfil diagnostic criteria for AD, but have been shown to have another pathological basis. These diseases are sometimes referred to as 'the real differential diagnosis of AD' and are listed in Table 1. In the following we will discuss some of them.

A depressive episode in the elderly may be accompanied by memory deficits. AD may, in turn, be accompanied by depression, thus making depression an important differential diagnostic consideration. Several studies have reported higher prevalence rates for signal hyperintensities in MRI in depressed

Table 1 *Differential diagnosis of 'probable' AD*

(Major) depression
Pick's disease
Frontal lobe dementia
Normal pressure hydrocephalus
Diffuse Lewy body disease
Posterior cortical atrophy
Primary progressive aphasia
Slowly progressive apraxia
Creutzfeld–Jakob disease
(Late onset) Huntington's disease

patients, suggesting a microvascular etiology for depression in late life (Brown *et al.*, 1992; Churchill *et al.*, 1992; Zubenko *et al.*, 1990). In the study of Zubenko *et al.* (1990) depressed patients showed the same amount of white matter changes on MRI as demented patients, but the latter group had significantly more cortical atrophy.

In Pick's disease and frontal lobe dementia usually a more focal pattern of atrophy is seen. A striking atrophy of the frontal lobes, sometimes with ballooning of the frontal horns, is usually seen (Figure 3), but sometimes a bilateral temporal lobe atrophy is found.

In normal pressure hydrocephalus (NPH) a typical picture of dilated ventricles without prominent cortical atrophy is seen. Often, MRI also shows a band of periventricular high signal intensity on the T2-weighted images, indicating transependymal CSF outflow (Figure 4). In more than 50% of such cases the etiology is unknown, although on neuropathological examination AD changes or vascular changes are often found. The pres-

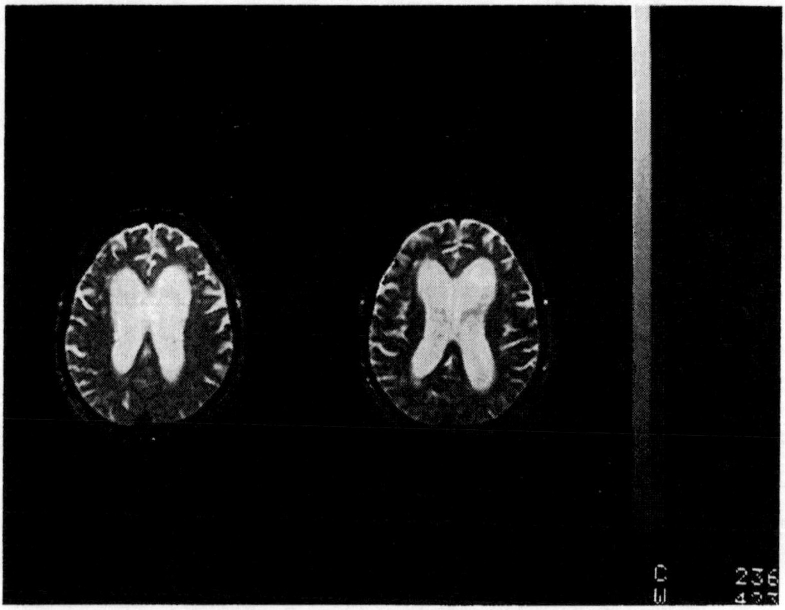

Figure 3 *Heavily T2-weighted axial MR images at two consecutive levels of a 66-year-old patient with a clinical diagnosis of frontal lobe dementia. Note the frontal cortical atrophy with widening of the frontal horns*

ence of severe medial temporal lobe atrophy on MRI may indicate co-existing AD, possibly predicting a poor shunt response with respect to cognitive functioning. The presence of a flow void (loss of signal intensity) in the aqueduct has been reported to be typical for NPH (Bradley *et al.*, 1991). However, this phenomenon has also been found in some other conditions. Quantitive measurements of the CSF flow through the aqueduct by means of cine-phase contrast MRI may be able to differentiate NPH cases from AD cases with enlarged ventricles, or may have a predictive value in selecting the right NPH candidates for a shunt.

'Diffuse Lewy body disease' may present with amnesia, aphasia, visuo-spatial disorientation and apraxia, complicated by hallucinations and confusion (Bordet and Destee, 1992). Extra-pyramidal features may occur in a later stage, as may be the case in AD. CT or MRI findings have been found not to be specific.

In cases of posterior cortical atrophy, as described by Benson *et al.* (1988), a prominent posterior atrophy with enlargement of the occipital horns is seen. Primary progressive aphasia (PPA) is

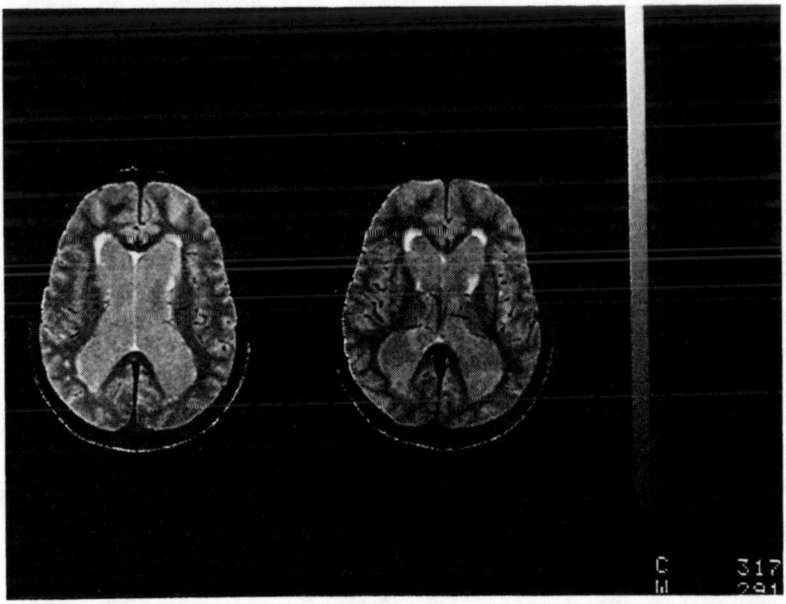

Figure 4 *Moderately T2-weighted axial MR images at two adjacent levels of a patient with a clinical diagnosis of NPH. Note the ventricular enlargement, widening of the corpus callosum angle and frontal 'caps'.*

a syndrome characterized by slowly progressive aphasia, usually non-fluent, of more than two years duration without subsequent development of dementia (Mesulam, 1982), although larger series have shown that some patients did become demented eventually (Mendez and Zander, 1991). Initial CT and MRI may show enlargement of the left Sylvian fissure. In advanced cases a bitemporal distribution of atrophy on MRI is described (Scheltens *et al.*, 1990, 1994a). Since aphasia may also be a presenting symptom of AD, it is important to predict whether PPA or AD will develop upon first presentation. In this context it has been suggested that absence of clear hippocampal atrophy on MRI is in favour of a diagnosis of PPA (De Boer *et al.*, 1992). Further studies with respect to these focal cortical syndromes are needed, since their neuropathological substrate may vary considerably, and may also include AD (Pogacar and Williams, 1984; Berthier *et al.*, 1991; Hof *et al.*, 1993).

Creutzfeld–Jakob disease may also be confused with AD, since myoclonus may accompany AD in a late stage and progression may be just as fast. Milton *et al.* (1991) and Tartaro *et al.* (1993) suggested that a diagnosis of Creutzfeld–Jakob disease has to be considered in a demented patient with basal ganglionic hyperintensity on MRI.

Finally, late onset Huntington's disease may occasionally present with memory disturbances in elderly patients, long before chorea becomes evident (Sax and Vonsattel, 1992). CT/MRI may show general brain atrophy and widening of the frontal parts of the lateral ventricles, indicating bilateral atrophy of the caudate nucleus, in advanced cases. Atrophy of the putamen, however, may be visible on MRI in an early stage (Bruyn *et al.*, 1993).

CT/MRI AND FUNCTIONAL STUDIES

It has been suggested that parietotemporal blood flow reduction may reflect pathological changes in the projection neurons in the parahippocampal gyrus, as found in monkeys (Mesulam *et al.*, 1977). Neurons that are pathologically affected in AD are predominantly projection neurons that interconnect association and limbic areas of the cortex, pyramidal neurons of the hippocampal formation and gyrus being especially affected. Medial temporal (hippocampal) atrophy in AD might follow the loss of these projection neurons. Thus, a combination of reduced parietotemporal blood flow and hippocampal atrophy might be highly specific for AD.

There have been two studies in which assessment of hippocampal atrophy on CT (Jobst *et al.*, 1992a) and MRI (Pearlson *et al.*, 1992) were combined with cerebral blood flow (SPECT) studies. In the study of Jobst *et al.* (1992a) linear measurements of medial temporal lobe atrophy were combined with ^{99}Tc-HMPAO SPECT to assess regional cerebral blood flow. The combination of hippocampal atrophy on CT and bitemporo-parietal hypoperfusion occurred in 44 of 51 AD patients, but only in two of 18 controls, and in four of 10 clinically non-Alzheimer-type demented patients, of whom one had necropsy evidence of AD. In another study, nine AD patients and eight control subjects underwent both MRI and ^{123}I-SPECT to detect regional cerebral blood flow changes (Pearlson *et al.*, 1992). Combining MRI and SPECT measures yielded 100% discrimination of the two groups. More recently we conducted a study in which we performed MRI and SPECT in a population randomly sampled from community dwelling elderly, as part of the longitudinal AMSTEL (Amsterdam Study of the Elderly) project (Launer *et al.*, 1993; Scheltens *et al.*, 1994b). In this study we found that hippocampal atrophy on MRI had a high sensitivity and specificity for AD, whereas SPECT did not. The positive predictive value of MRI was modest (41%) but the negative predictive value was high (91%). Moreover, combining MRI and SPECT resulted in a decrease of both sensitivity and specificity. Our results stress that a diagnostic test has to be tested in a sample representative of the general population in order to establish sensitivity and specificity values. It nicely demonstrates that the results may then be less impressive than expected (Sackett *et al.*, 1985).

CONCLUSIONS

Based on the reviewed literature it becomes clear that for the exclusion of other causes of dementia CT may be used. Finding cortical or subcortical atrophy on CT or MRI itself does not indicate AD, unless an increase in CSF volume over a period of one year is documented. Reviewing the available data on hippocampal atrophy on CT/MRI, one is inclined to speculate that it provides a useful early marker. CT and MRI based measurements of hippocampal atrophy show promise in providing useful diagnostic information for separating patients with probable AD from normal elderly individuals. The use of a standardized imaging protocol, including some assessment of hippocampal atrophy, can be considered a cost-effective approach. In the evaluation of patients with dementia, they must undergo a cross-sectional imaging study to exclude other (treatable) causes of dementia. For scientific studies, volumetric measurements will be mandatory, because of the incorporation of adjustment for age and intracranial volume. This is best done on MRI. However, in clinical practice, simple visual inspection, using either CT or MRI, may provide the clinician with ample diagnostic information with respect to the presence of AD. As shown above, visual assessment yields similar sensitivity on CT and MRI. Combining either assessment of hippocampal atrophy with cerebral blood flow measurements on SPECT does not seem to be warranted both from a clinical and economical point of view.

REFERENCES

Albert, M., Naeser, M. A., Levine, H. L., and Garvey, A. J. (1984a) CT density numbers in patients with senile dementia of Alzheimer's type. *Arch. Neurol.*, **41**, 1264–1269.

Albert, M., Naeser, M. A., Levine, H. L., and Garvey, A. J. (1984b) Ventricular size in patients with presenile dementia of the Alzheimer's type. *Arch Neurol.*, **41**, 1258–1263.

Altshuler, L. L., Casanova, M. F., Goldberg, T. E., and Kleinman, J. E. (1990) The hippocampus and parahippocampus in schizophrenic, suicide and control brains. *Arch. Gen. Psychiatry*, **47**, 1029–1034.

American Psychiatric Association (1987) *Diagnostic and Statistical Manual of Mental Disorders*, 3rd rev. edn. American Psychiatric Association, Washington DC, pp. 103–107.

Ball, M. J., Fisman, M., Hachinski, V., *et al.* (1985) A new definition of Alzheimer's disease: a hippocampal dementia. *Lancet*, **i**, 14–16.

Baxter, B. S., and Sorenson, J. A. (1981) Factors affecting the measurement of size and CT number in computed tomography. *Invest. Radiol.*, **16**, 337–341.

Benson, D. F., Davis, R. J., and Snyder, B. D. (1988) Posterior cortical atrophy. *Arch. Neurol.*, **45**, 789–793.

Berthier, M. L., Leiguarda, R., Starkstein, S. E., Sevlever, G., and Taratuto, A. L. (1991) Alzheimer's disease in a patient with posterior cortical atrophy. *J. Neurol. Neurosurg. Psychiatry*, **54**, 1110–1111.

Bhatia, S., Bookheimer, S. Y., Gaillard, W. D., and Theodore, W. H. (1993) Measurement of whole temporal lobe and hippocampus for MR volumetry. Normative data. *Neurology*, **43**, 2006–2010.

Bordet, R., and Destee, A. (1992) De la maladie de Parkinson à la maladie des corps de Lewy. *Presse Méd.*, **21**, 708–712.

Braak, H., Braak, E., and Bohl, J. (1993) Staging of Alzheimer related cortical destruction. *Eur. Neurol.*, **33**, 403–408.

Bradley, W. G. Jr, Whittemore, A. R., Watanabe, A. S., Davis, A. J., Teresi, L. M., and Homyak, M. (1991) Association of deep white matter infarction with chronic communicating hydrocephalus: implications regarding the possible origin of normal pressure hydrocephalus. *AJNR*, **12**, 31–39.

Brinkman, S. D., Sarwar, M., Levin, H. S., and Morris, H. H. (1981) Quantitative indexes of computed tomography in dementia and normal aging. *Radiology*, **138**, 89–92.

Brinkman, S. D., and Largen, J. W. (1984) Changes in brain ventricular size with repeated CAT scans in suspected Alzheimer's disease. *Am. J. Psychiatry*, **141**, 81–83.

Brown, F. W., Lewine, R. J., Hudgins, P. A., and Risch, S. C. (1992) White matter hyperintense signals in psychiatric and nonpsychiatric subjects. *Am. J. Psychiatry*, **149**, 620–625.

Bruyn, R. P. M., Hageman, G. A., Geelen, J. A. G., *et al.* (1993) SPECT, CT and MRI investigations of a Turkish family with Huntington's disease. *Neuroradiology*, **35**, 525–528.

Churchill, C. M., Priolo, C. V., Nemeroff, C. B., Krishnan, R. R., and Breitner, J. (1992) Occult subcortical magnetic resonance findings in elderly depressives. *Int. J. Geriatr. Psychiatry*, **16**, 213–216.

Cuenod, C. A., Denys, A., Michot, J. L., Jehenson, P., Forrette, F., Kaplan, D., Syrota, A., and Boller, F. (1993) Amygdala atrophy in Alzheimer's disease. An in vivo magnetic resonance imaging study. *Arch. Neurol.*, **50**, 941–945.

Damasio, A. R., Eslinger, P. J., Damasio, H., Van Hoesen, G. W., and Cornell, S. (1985) Multimodel amnesic syndrome following bilateral temporal and basal forebrain damage. *Arch. Neurol.*, **42**, 252–259.

De Boer, M., Wolters, E. Ch., and Scheltens, Ph. (1992) Slowly progressive aphasia without dementia: differentiation from Alzheimer's disease by means of Magnetic Resonance Imaging. *Neurobiol. Aging*, **13**(suppl. 1), S22.

De Carli, C., Kaye, J. A., Horwitz, B., and Rapoport, S. (1990) Critical analysis of the use of computer-assisted transverse axial tomography to study human brain aging and dementia of the Alzheimer type. *Neurology*, **40**, 872–883.

De Carli, C., Haxby, J. V., Gillette, J. A., Teichberg, D., Rapoport, S. I., and Schapiro, M. B. (1992) Longitudinal changes in lateral ventricular volume in patients with dementia of the Alzheimer type. *Neurology*, **42**, 2029–2036.

De Leon, M. J., George, A. E., Reisberg, B., *et al.* (1989a) Alzheimer's disease: longitudinal CT studies of ventricular change. *AJNR*, **10**, 371–376.

De Leon, M. J., George, A. E., Stylopoulos, L. A., Smith, G., and Miller, D. C. (1989b) Early marker for Alzheimer's disease: the atrophic hippocampus. *Lancet*, **ii**, 672–673.

De Leon, M. J., Smith, G., Convit, A., *et al.* (1992) The early detection of brain pathology in Alzheimer's disease. In Y. Christen and P. Churchland (eds), *Neurophilosophy and Alzheimer's Disease*. Springer-Verlag, Berlin.

De Leon, M. J., Golomb, J., Convit, A., De Santi, S., McRae, Th. D., and George, A. E. (1993) Measurement of medial temporal lobe atrophy in diagnosis of Alzheimer's disease. *Lancet*, **341**, 125.

Drayer, B. P. (1988) Imaging of the aging brain. Part 1. Normal findings. *Radiology*, **166**, 785–796.

Engel, P. A., and Gelber, J. (1992) Does computed tomographic brain imaging have a place in the diagnosis of dementia? *Arch. Intern. Med.*, **152**, 1437–1440.

Erkinjuntti, T., Lee, D. H., Gao, F., Steenhuis, R., Eliasziw, M., Fry, R., Merskey, H., and Hachinski, V. C. (1993) Temporal lobe atrophy on magnetic resonance imaging in the diagnosis of early Alzheimer's disease. *Arch. Neurol.*, **50**, 305–310.

Folstein, M. F., Folstein, S. E. and McHugh, P. R. (1975) Mini Mental State: a practical method for grading the cognitive state of patients for the clinician. *J. Psychiatr. Res.*, **12**, 189–198.

Gado, M., Hughes, C. P., Danziger, W., Chi, D., Jost, G., and Berg, L. (1982) Volumetric measurements of the cerebrospinal fluid spaces in demented subjects and controls. *Radiology*, **144**, 535–538.

George, A. E., De Leon, M. J., Stylopoulos, L. A. *et al.* (1990) CT diagnostic features of Alzheimer disease: importance of the choroidal/hippocampal fissure complex. *AJNR*, **11**, 101–107.

Golomb, J., De Leon, M. J., Kluger, A., George, A. E., Tarshish, C., and Ferris, S. H. (1993) Hippocampal atrophy in normal aging. An association with recent memory impairment. *Arch. Neurol.*, **50**, 967–973.

Hof, P. R., Archin, N., Osmand, A. P., Doughertry, J. H., Wells, C., Bouras, C., and Morrison, J. H. (1993) Posterior cortical atrophy in Alzheimer's disease: analysis of a new case and re-evaluation of a historical report. *Acta Neuropathol.*, **86**, 215–223.

Ikeda, M., Tanabe, H., Nakagawa, Y., Kazui, H., Oi, H., Yamazaki, H., Harada, K., and Nishimura, T. (1994) MRI based quantitative assessment of the hippocampal region in very mild to moderate Alzheimer's disease. *Neuroradiology*, **36**, 7–10.

Jack, C. R. Jr, Sharbrough, F. W., Cascino, G. D., Hirschorn, K. A., O'Brien, P. C., and Marsh, W. R. (1992a) Magnetic resonance image-based hippocampal volumetry: correlation with outcome after temporal lobectomy. *Ann. Neurol.*, **31**, 138–146.

Jack, C. R. Jr, Petersen, R. C., O'Brien, P. C., and Tangalos, E. G. (1992b) MR-based hippocampal volumetry in the diagnosis of Alzheimer's disease. *Neurology*, **42**, 183–188.

Jacoby, R. J., Levy, R., and Dawson, J. M. (1980a) Computed tomography in the elderly: I. The normal population. *Br. J. Psychiatry*, **136**, 249–255.

Jacoby, R. J., Levy, R., and Dawson, J. M. (1980b) Computed tomography in the elderly. II. Senile dementia: diagnosis and functional impairment. *Br. J. Psychiatry*, **136**, 256–269.

Jellinger, K. (1990) Morphology of Alzheimer's disease and related disorders. In K. Maurer, H. Beckmann and P. Riederer (eds), *Alzheimer's Disease. Epidemiology, Neuropathology, Neurochemistry, and Clinics.* Vienna: Springer, pp. 61–77.

Jobst, K. A., Smith, A. D., and Barker, C. S. (1992a) Association of atrophy of the medial temporal lobe with reduced blood flow in the posterior parietotemporal cortex in patients with a clinical and pathological diagnosis of Alzheimer's disease. *J. Neurol. Neurosurg. Psychiatry*, **55**, 190–194.

Jobst, K. A., Smith, A. D., Szatmari, M. *et al.* (1992b) Detection in life of confirmed Alzheimer's disease using a simple measurement of medial temporal lobe atrophy by computed tomography. *Lancet*, **340**, 1179–1183.

Kesslak, J. P., Nalcioglu, O., and Cotman, C. W. (1991) Quantification of magnetic resonance scans for hippocampal and parahippocampal atrophy in Alzheimer's disease. *Neurology*, **41**, 51–54.

Kido, D. K., Cain, E. D., Lemay, M., Ekholm, S., Booth, H., and Panzer, R. (1989) Temporal lobe atrophy in patients with Alzheimer disease: a CT study. *AJNR*, **10**, 551–555.

Killiany, R. J., Moss, M. B., Albert, M. S., Sandor, T., Tieman, J., and Jolesz, F. (1993) Temporal lobe regions on magnetic resonance imaging identify patients with early Alzheimer's disease. *Arch. Neurol.*, **50**, 949–954.

Kukull, W. A., Larson, E. B., Reifler, B. V., Lampe, T. H., Yerby, M., and Hughes, J. (1990) Interrater reliability of Alzheimer's disease diagnosis. *Neurology*, **40**, 257–260.

Laffey, P. A., Peyster, R. G., Nathan, R., Huskin, M. E., and McGinley, J. A. (1984) Computed tomography and aging: results in a normal elderly population. *Neuroradiology*, **26**, 273–278.

Launer, L. J., Dinkgreve, M., Jonker, C., *et al.* (1993) Are age and education independent correlates of the Mini-Mental state exam performance of community dwelling elderly? *J. Gerontol.*, **48**, 271–277.

LeMay, M., Stafford, J. L., Sandor, T., Albert, M., Haykal, H., and Zamani, A. (1986) Statistical assessment of perceptual CT scan ratings in patients with Alzheimer type dementia. *J. Comput. Assist. Tomogr.*, **10**, 802–809.

Leys, D., Pruvo, J. P., Petit, H., Gaudet, Y., and Clarisse, J. (1989) Maladie d'Alzheimer. Analyse statistique des résultats du scanner X. *Rev. Neurol. (Paris)*, **145**, 134–139.

Leys, D., Pruvo, J. P., and Petit, H. (1990) Changes in cerebral atrophy with repeated CT scans: a useful tool to predict further Alzheimer's disease? *J. Neurol.*, **237**, S105.

Lopez, O. L., Swihart, A. A., Becker, J.T., *et al.* (1990) Reliability of NINCDS-ADRDA clinical criteria for the diagnosis of Alzheimer's disease. *Neurology*, **40**, 1517–1522.

Luxenberg, J. S., Haxby, J. V., Creasey, H., Sundaram, M., and Rapoport, S. I. (1987) Rate of ventricular enlargement in dementia of the Alzheimer type correlates with rate of neuropsychological deterioration. *Neurology*, **37**, 1135–1140.

McKhann, G., Drachman, D., Folstein, M., Katzman, R., Price, D., and Stadlan, E. M. (1984) Clinical diagnosis of Alzheimer's disease: report of NINCDS-ADRDA work group under the auspices of Department of Health and Human Services Task Force on Alzheimer's disease. *Neurology*, **34**, 939–944

Mendez, M. F., and Zander, B. A. (1991) Dementia presenting with aphasia: clinical characteristics. *J. Neurol. Neurosurg. Psychiatry*, **54**, 542–545.

Mesulam, M. M. (1982) Slowly progressive aphasia without generalized dementia. *Ann. Neurol.*, **11**, 592–598.

Mesulam, M. M., Van Hoesen, G.W., Pandya, D. N., *et al.* (1977) Limbic and sensory connections of the inferior parietal lobule (area PG) in the rhesus monkey: a study with a new method for horseradish peroxidase histochemistry. *Brain Res.*, **136**, 393–414.

Milton, W. J., Atlas, S. W., Lavi, E., and Mollman, J. E. (1991) Magnetic resonance imaging of Creutzfeldt–Jakob disease. *Ann. Neurol.*, **29**, 438–440.

Pearlson, G. D., Harris, G., Powers, R. E., *et al.* (1992) Quantitative changes in mesial temporal volume, regional cerebral blood flow, and cognition in Alzheimer's disease. *Arch. Gen. Psychiatry*, **49**, 402–408.

Penn, R. D., Belanger, M. G., and Yasnoff, W. A. (1978) Ventricular volume in man computed from CAT scans. *Ann. Neurol.*, **3**, 216–233.

Philbot, M., and Burns, A. (1993) Jobst *et al.*'s 'Detection in life of confirmed Alzheimer's disease using a simple measurement of medial temporal lobe atrophy by computed tomography'. *Br. J. Psychiatry*, **163**, 809–812.

Pogacar, S., and Williams, R. S. (1984) Alzheimer's disease presenting as slowly progressive aphasia. *RI Med. J.*, **67**, 181–185.

Press, G. A., Amaral, D. G., and Squire, L. R. (1989) Hippocampal abnormalities in amnesic patients revealed by high-resolution magnetic resonance imaging. *Nature*, **341**, 54–57.

Rusinek, H., De Leon, M. J., George, A. E., *et al.* (1991) Alzheimer disease: measuring loss of cerebral gray matter with MR imaging. *Radiology*, **178**, 109–114.

Sackett, D. L., Haynes, R. B., and Tugwell, P. (1985) *Clinical Epidemiology. A Basic Science for Clinical Medicine.* Boston/Toronto: Little, Brown.

Sandor, T., Albert, M., Stafford, J., and Harpley, J. S. (1988) Discrimination of Alzheimer patients and normal controls using a computerized CT analysis. *AJNR*, **9**, 1181–1187.

Sandor, T., Jolesz, F., Tieman, J., Kikinis, R., Jones, K., and Albert, M (1992) Comparative analysis of computed tomographic and magnetic resonance imaging scans in Alzheimer patients and controls. *Arch. Neurol.*, **49**, 381–384.

Sax, D. S., and Vonsattel, J–P. (1992) Chorea and progressive dementia in an 88-year old woman. *N. Engl. J. Med.*, **326**, 117–125.

Scheltens, Ph., Hazenberg, G. J., Lindeboom, J., Valk, J., and Wolters, E. Ch. (1990) A case of progressive aphasia without dementia: 'temporal' Pick's disease? *J. Neurol. Neurosurg. Psychiatry*, **53**, 79–80.

Scheltens, Ph., Leys, D., Barkhof, F., *et al.* (1992a) Atrophy of the medial temporal lobes on MRI in Alzheimer's disease and normal aging. Diagnostic value and neuropsychological correlates. *J. Neurol. Neurosurg. Psychiatry*, **55**, 967–972.

Scheltens, Ph., Weinstein, H., and Van Gool, W. A. (1992b) De waarde van de nieuwe diagnostische technieken bij de ziekte van Alzheimer. *Ned. Tijdschr. Geneeskd.*, **136**, 2459–2462.

Scheltens, Ph., Ravid, R., and Kamphorst, W. (1994a) Pathologic findings in a case of primary progressive aphasia. *Neurology*, **44**, 279–282.

Scheltens, Ph., Launer, L. J., Barkhof, F., Weinstein, H.C., and Jonker, C. (1994b) The value of magnetic resonance imaging and single photon emission computed tomography in the diagnosis of Alzheimer's disease in an unselected elderly population. *Neurology*, **44**, A179.

Schmidt, R. (1992) Comparison of magnetic resonance imaging in Alzheimer's disease, vascular dementia and normal aging. *Eur. Neurol.*, **32**, 164–169.

Scoville, W. B., and Milner, B. (1957) Loss of recent memory after bilateral hippocampal lesions. *J. Neurol. Neurosurg. Psychiatry*, **20**, 11–21.

Seab, J. P., Jagust, W. J., Wong, S. T. S., Roos, M. S., Reed, B. R., and Budinger, T. P. (1988) Quantitative NMR measurements of hippocampal atrophy in Alzheimer's disease. *Magn. Reson. Med.*, **8**, 200–208.

Sullivan, E. V., Shear, P. K., Mathalon, D. H., Lim, K. O., Yesavage, J. A., Tinklenberg, J. R., and Pfefferbaum, A. (1993) Greater abnormalities of brain cerebrospinal fluid volumes in younger than in older patients with Alzheimer's disease. *Arch. Neurol.*, **50**, 359–373.

Takeda, S., and Matsuzawa, T. (1985a) Age-related change in volumes of the ventricles, cisternae and sulci: a quantitative study using computed tomography. *J. Am. Geriatr. Soc.*, **33**, 264–268.

Takeda, S., and Matsuzawa, T. (1985b) Age-related brain atrophy: a study with computed tomography. *J. Gerontol.*, **40**, 159–163.

Tanna, N. K., Kohn, M. I., Horwich, D. N., *et al.* (1991) Analysis of brain and cerebrospinal fluid volumes with MR imaging: impact on PET data correction for atrophy. *Radiology*, **178**, 123–130.

Tartaro, A., Fulgente, T., Pizzi, C. D., Bonomo, L., Bocola, V., and Onofrj, M. (1993) MRI alterations as an early finding in Creutzfeld Jakob disease. *Eur. J. Radiol.*, **17**, 155–158.

Tierney, M. C., Fisher, R. H., Lewis, A. J., *et al.* (1988) The NINCDS-ADRDA work group criteria for the clinical diagnosis of probable Alzheimer's disease: a clinicopathologic study of 57 cases. *Neurology*, **38**, 359–364.

Tomlinson, B. E., Blessed, G., and Roth, M. (1968) Observations on the brains of non-demented old people. *J. Neurol. Sci.*, **7**, 331–356.

Turkheimer, E., Cullum, C. M., Hubler, D. W., Paver, S. W., Yeo, R. A., and Bigler, E. D. (1984) Quantifying cortical atrophy. *J. Neurol. Neurosurg. Psychiatry*, **47**, 1314–1318.

Valk, J., and van der Knaap, M. S. (1989) *Magnetic Resonance of Myelin, Myelination and Myelin Disorders*. Springer-Verlag, Berlin.

Willmer, J., Carruthers, A., Guzaman, D. A., Collins, B., Pogue, J., and Stuss, D. T. (1993) The usefulness of CT scanning in diagnosing dementia of the Alzheimer type. *Can. J. Neurol. Sci.*, **20**, 210–216.

Zatz, L. M., Jernigan, T. L., and Ahumada, A. J. (1982) Changes on computed cranial tomography with aging: intracranial fluid volume. *AJNR*, **3**, 1–11.

Zatz, L. M., and Jernigan, T. L. (1983) The ventricular–brain ratio on computed tomography scans: validity and proper use. *Psychiatry Res.*, **8**, 207–214.

Zola-Morgan, S., Squire, L. R., and Amaral, D. G. (1986) Human amnesia and the medial temporal region. Enduring memory impairment following a bilateral lesion limited to field CA1 of the hippocampus. *J. Neurosci.*, **6**, 2950–2967.

Zubenko, G. S., Sullivan, P., Nelson, J. P., Belle, S. H., Huff, J., and Wolf, G. L. (1990) Brain imaging abnormalities in mental disorders of late life. *Arch. Neurol.*, **47**, 1107–1111.

4

The Cholinergic Hypothesis in Alzheimer's Disease—Clinical Evidence Gained with Velnacrine[1]

K. Siegfried

Clinical Research Department, Hoechst AG, Frankfurt am Main, Germany

ABSTRACT

Increased research efforts in the 1970s/early 1980s brought about evidence of a significant deficit in the level of the neurotransmitter acetylcholine in brains of patients with Alzheimer's disease (AD). As a consequence, clinical researchers tested the effects of cholinergic agents on cognitive core symptoms of AD. Of the drugs initially selected, physostigmine, a cholinesterase inhibitor, showed the best results. The effects were, however, only short-lasting and generally very mild. Therefore, a group of new cholinesterase inhibitors, the aminoacridines (velnacrine, tacrine), was developed in the hope of overcoming these

[1] This chapter gives a survey of both US and European results obtained with velnacrine. The author thanks his US colleagues from Clinical Neuroscience/ Hoechst-Roussel Pharmaceuticals, Inc. (Drs R. Allen, M. F. Murphy, R. Civil, and F. J. Huff) for providing him with the US results.

Alzheimer's Disease: Clinical and Treatment Perspectives. Edited by N. R. Cutler, C. G. Gottfries and K. Siegfried.

weaknesses. The present chapter reviews data from phase II and III clinical trials with velnacrine. The conclusion is that these types of drugs are efficacious and appear to have clinically relevant effects in a subgroup of patients with AD. They also have some obvious safety problems, mainly transaminase increases, which seem to be acceptable provided certain precautions are observed. An important limitation of the aminoacridines is the lack of diagnostic tools to identify the subgroup of potential responders. The obvious pharmacological heterogeneity of patients with AD requires an improved diagnostic classification system and reliable tools for patient subtyping.

INTRODUCTION

Alzheimer's disease (AD) is a primary degenerative disease characterized by a steadily progressive intellectual deterioration. Alois Alzheimer, who first described this disease in 1906 at a symposium of German psychiatrists and neurologists and published the description in 1907 in the *Zentralblatt für Neurologie und Psychiatrie*, volume 18 (Alzheimer, 1907; Wilkins and Brody, 1969; Hoff and Hippius, 1989), considered it as a presenile type of dementia (i.e. with occurrence in patients under 65 years of age), distinct from senile forms. In the 1970s, however, various research groups, mainly in the USA, emphasized that histopathologic brain changes in the senile and presenile forms appear to be virtually indistinguishable. Therefore, both groups were combined under the label 'Alzheimer's disease' (AD) (Cohen, 1983; McKhann *et al.*, 1984). Although the question as to whether AD represents one or several diseases has remained a controversial issue (Gottfries, 1989, 1993; Blennow, 1990; Wilcock, 1991; Gottfries *et al.*, Chapter 1), the merge of the presenile and senile forms tremendously stimulated research activities because of the high relative frequency of the senile form and the increasing proportion of elderly people in Western societies. Prevalence rates of moderate and severe dementia exponentially increase with aging from 3 to 5% in the age-group of 65 to 70 years and double approximately with every five years of age to 25 to 30% of the population beyond the age of 80. Approximately 60% of these dementias are attributed to AD (Haefner, 1989).

The initial finding of systematic research efforts in the 1970s and early 1980s was evidence of a significant deficit in the level of the neurotransmitter acetylcholine in brains of patients with AD. This led to the hypothesis that AD is characterized by a specific neurotransmitter pathology, a central cholinergic deficit, which seems to underly the essential cognitive deficiencies of this type of dementia (Bartus *et al.*, 1985; Perry, 1987; Siegfried, 1992; Siegfried and Murphy, 1993). The most important evidence in favor of the hypothesis were postmortem findings which showed significantly (by 40–90%) reduced activity of choline acetyltransferase (CAT) in the brains of patients with AD in comparison with age-matched controls (Davies, 1981; Perry *et al.*, 1977). CAT is an enzyme which produces and releases in neurons the neurotransmitter acetylcholine. Pharmacological studies showed that scopolamine, a centrally active anticholinergic agent, caused both in animals and humans typical deteriorations of attentional and recent memory functions which resembled the cognitive dysfunction in early stages of AD. This dysfunction could, again, be improved or reversed by the administration of the centrally active cholinesterase inhibitor physostigmine (Drachman and Leavitt, 1974; Davis *et al.*, 1981; Christie *et al.*, 1981). Of special importance was evidence that the amount of cholinergic abnormalities correlates on the one hand with the number of senile plaques in the brains of patients with AD and, on the other, with mental test scores obtained from these patients shortly before their death (Perry *et al.*, 1978).

Meanwhile the efficacy of physostigmine in patients with AD has been tested by several separate clinical research teams (Beller *et al.*, 1985; Blackwood and Christie, 1986; Agnoli *et al.*, 1983; Caltagirone *et al.*, 1982; Davidson *et al.*, 1986; Davis and Mohs, 1982). The majority of studies were able to demonstrate some improvement, but the effects were not of clinical relevance. They varied considerably amongst patients, possibly owing to large variations in the bioavailability of the drug, and were generally small and short-lasting. The latter could have been expected in view of the short elimination half-life (approx. 20 min) of the drug. Finally, there was a very small safety margin between effective doses and those which caused marked peripheral cholinergic side-effects (e.g. vomiting, diarrhea). The conclusion was that for an effective treatment of AD a compound was needed that would have a similar biochemical mode of action like physostigmine (i.e. cholinesterase inhibition) but a better bioavailability and longer elimination half-life. It was hoped that these pharmacokinetic properties would result in clinically more relevant effects. The remaining part of this chapter will deal with the question if these assumptions and conclusions were correct and helped to find a successful treatment for patients with AD.

DECISIVE QUESTIONS FOR EVALUATING THE USEFULNESS OF THE CHOLINERGIC TREATMENT APPROACH

The usefulness of the cholinergic approach in the treatment of AD will be discussed by trying to answer the following clinically important questions:

- Is there evidence for the efficacy of the cholinergic treatment in patients with AD?
- What is the onset of action and the duration of effects in the treatment of these patients? In particular, is there evidence of sustained effects?
- Which are the target symptoms of a cholinergic treatment?
- Is the effect size sufficient?
- Are the effects clinically relevant?
- Is the risk–benefit ratio of the first effective AD agents, the aminoacridines, acceptable?
- What are the limitations of the cholinergic treatment approach?

An answer to these questions will be attempted by reviewing evidence from clinical studies with velnacrine in patients with AD. Velnacrine is a 1,2,3,4-tetrahydro-9-aminoacridine-1-ol maleate and acts as a potent cholinesterase inhibitor with marked central nervous effects. It is chemically related to tacrine. Pharmacological studies with velnacrine have demonstrated that it enhances memory and learning functions and can reverse disturbances of these functions caused by cholinergic deficits (Fielding *et al.*, 1989). In pharmacokinetic studies in healthy young and elderly subjects (Puri *et al.*, 1988), peak plasma levels were reached within one hour after oral administration and the elimination half-life was between 2 and 3 hours. The absorption and amount of drug excreted proved to be dose-related. Steady-state plasma levels were reached after three days of repeated (t.i.d) oral administration. In the elderly, peak plasma levels and the amount of absorption tend to be higher and elimination half-life longer than in young subjects. The velnacrine studies reviewed here were carried out in patients with mild to moderately severe degrees of 'probable AD' according to NINCDS-ADRDA criteria (McKhann *et al.*, 1984). The severity of the disease was primarily determined by the Folstein Mini-Mental Scale (FMMS scores 10–24; in case of initially high intellectual level: 27) (Folstein *et al.*, 1975). The most important exclusion criteria were: dementias of another origin, e.g. due to vitamin B12 and folic acid deficiencies, hypothyroidism, cerebral trauma, neoplasms, normal pressure hydrocephalus, vascular factors (criteria: scores of >4 on the modified Hachinski Ischemia Scale: Rosen *et al.*, 1980; stepwise deteriorating course of the disease rather than uniformly progressive deterioration; mass lesions on CAT scan), and 'pseudodementia' (due to major psychiatric diseases). Also excluded were patients with major concomitant (cardiovascular, respiratory, hepatic, renal, and hematologic) diseases. The review is based on a total number of approximately 1500 patients treated with velnacrine.

EVIDENCE OF EFFICACY IN PATIENTS WITH MILD TO MODERATELY SEVERE DEGREES OF AD

Evidence of efficacy for velnacrine comes from four double-blind placebo-controlled studies which are listed below (Table 1). These studies varied in the number of patients treated, the duration of treatment, and the study design used.

In spite of variations in design, number of patients treated and treatment duration, all four studies consistently showed efficacy of velnacrine over placebo:

- In the European early phase II pilot study (2 times 10 day cross-over) there was a significant treatment effect ($p = 0.013$)

Table 1 *Evidence of efficacy for velnacrine in patients with AD*

Phase of development	Study number	Study design	Duration of treatment*	Sample size†
Early phase II (Pilot)	202DZ (Europe)	Double-blind placebo-controlled cross-over	2 × 10 days	45 patients (34 patients)
Late phase II	201USA	Enrichment procedure (main segment: double-blind placebo-controlled)	13 weeks (6 weeks)	735 patients (309 patients)
Phase III	301DZ (Europe)	Enrichment procedure (main segment: double-blind placebo-controlled parallel group comparison)	26 weeks (4 months)	239 patients (114 patients)
Phase III	301USA	Double-blind placebo-controlled parallel-group comparison	6 months	449 patients

* Duration of treatment: The figures without brackets give the treatment duration of the total study whereas figures in brackets indicate the duration of double-blind parallel-group treatment.

† Number of patients: Figures in brackets indicate the number of patients in the main (parallel-group) study segment.

on the cognitive behavior subscale (without memory tasks) of the Alzheimer Disease Assessment Scale (ADAS: Rosen *et al.*, 1984), in a computerized Word Recognition Task ($p = 0.048$) (Wesnes, 1985), in an aggregate measure (of days 1, 4, and 10 of each treatment phase) of the Clinical Impression of Change Rating (CGI-Ch.) (NIMH, 1976), and a Choice Reaction Time Task ($p = 0.002$) (Wesnes, 1985).

- In the phase II US enrichment study, after six weeks of double-blind parallel-group treatment (main study segment) there was a significant effect, compared to placebo, on the ADAS Cognitive Score (comprised of cognitive items and memory tasks) ($p = 0.001$) and on the CGI-Change Rating ($p = 0.046$).
- At the end of the four-month double-blind placebo-controlled treatment of the main study segment of the European phase III enrichment study (Scheltens *et al.*, 1994), the results significantly favored velnacrine on the ADAS Cognitive Subscale ($p = 0.038$). Presumably due to complications inherent in the enrichment procedure (e.g. shifting baselines), the Clinical

Global Impression of Change Rating did not become significant. (Similar problems were encountered in the tacrine enrichment study: Davis *et al.*, 1992.) Significant effects were also observed on the following secondary outcome variables: carers' ratings on the subscales 'Memory' ($p = 0.04$) and 'Instrumental Activities of Daily Living' ($p = 0.04$) of the 'Nurses Observation Geriatric Scale' (NOSGER: Spiegel, 1989), Digit Symbol Substitution Test ($p = 0.04$) (Wechsler, 1958), Paired-Associate Learning Task ($p = 0.04$ (Inglis, 1959).

- Finally, the phase III US study, which was a six-month double-blind placebo-controlled parallel-group trial (without an enrichment procedure), was able to confirm the above-mentioned results: The completer analysis after six months of treatment brought about significant effects for velnacrine over placebo on the ADAS Cognitive Subscale ($p = 0.05$), the CGI-Change ($p = 0.05$), and carers' ratings on the 'Patient Global Improvement Rating' (PGIR; $p = 0.005$) and the 'Physical Self-Maintenance Scale' (PSMS; $p = 0.026$). The Last Observation Carried Forward Analyses (which do not only include completers but also the last assessments of drop-outs) generally rendered even more favorable p-values.

In summary, there was a marked degree of consistency in the efficacy results:

- Consistency of the four studies: all of them rendered significant results in favor of velnacrine on more than two efficacy variables.
- Consistency of the results of different assessment methods (i.e. comprehensive clinical scale of cognitive core symptoms of AD; clinical global ratings; carers' ratings of behavior in everyday life; cognitive performance tests).
- Consistency of results coming from different (and separate) observers: clinicians (clinical global impression ratings), psychometricians (ADAS cognitive subscale and cognitive performance tests), and carers (NOSGER, Physical Self-Maintenance Scale, Global Impression Rating).

The most recent (5th) draft edition of the European Guidelines on Antidementia Compounds (CPMP, 1992) considers the consistency of the results of different outcome measures obtained by separate observers, as decisive evidence of efficacy.

ONSET OF ACTION AND THE DURATION OF EFFECTS

Knowledge about the onset of action of a treatment is of clinical importance because it will determine when the clinician can reasonably make a judgement about response. The earlier such a decision can be made the quicker a patient who is unlikely to profit from a drug can be discontinued from treatment and is thus no longer exposed to an unnecessary risk of adverse events.

Significant effects of a single dose of 75 mg of velnacrine over both placebo and physostigmine (2 mg p.o.) were observed in patients with AD as early as two hours after drug administration on a simple word recognition task (Ebmeier *et al.*, 1992; Siegfried, 1993a, 1993b). These effects were, however, quite subtle. A longer treatment duration is needed to observe more pronounced early effects which can be obtained in clinical observations: in the phase II US enrichment study (201USA), decisions about patients' response were based on one-week treatment periods; the European cross-over trial (202DZ) showed significant effects after 10 days of treatment, and the European phase III enrichment study (301MN) used a three-week 'test treatment' with velnacrine (50 mg t.i.d) successfully to make a judgement on patients' response. In all of these trials, the Clinical Global Impression of Change Rating correlated with the ADAS response criterion (i.e. at least a 4-point improvement on the ADAS cognitive subscale). Patients meeting this criterion were on average rated as 'minimally or moderately improved'. Response after one month of treatment correlated significantly ($r = 0.49$; $p = 0.0001$; $n = 52$) with changes observed after four months (endpoint) (Scheltens *et al.*, 1994). The conclusion is that velnacrine has a fairly early onset of action. Depending on the titration schedule used (i.e. speed of dose escalation up to the highest dose of 75 mg t.i.d.), the adequate duration of a test treat-ment for a clinical evaluation of response ranges from approximately three to six weeks.

In a progressive disease like AD which requires chronic treatment, the question of sustained treatment effects is of particular relevance. The results of the above-mentioned four and six-month double-blind placebo-controlled treatment studies showed that velnacrine was at endpoint still significantly superior to placebo. Patients were on average still found improved in comparison to baseline whereas placebo patients had deteriorated. Another piece of evidence for sustained effects comes from clinical global impression ratings obtained during open-labelled treatment extension. In the fourth quarter of 1993, slightly more than 100 patients, who came from various study protocols, had a treatment extension of more than one year, 95 of whom were eligible for efficacy evaluation. After one year of treatment extension, patients received the following evaluations on the Clinical Global Impression Ratings of Change: 43.2% were rated as (still) improved in comparison to baseline, 37.8% as not changed, and only 19.0% as impaired. In order to interpret these figures adequately, one has to take into account the progressive downhill course of AD which, as a rule, brings about a marked deterioration in most of the (untreated) patients after a period of six to twelve months. In summary, there is evidence of sustained effects of velnacrine. The data suggest an approximately six to twelve-month retardation of the progression of the disease. Similar observations have been made with tacrine (Holford and Peace, 1992). Further methodologically more rigorous studies of ≥12 months duration are needed to confirm this clinical impression. In addition, it would be useful to identify patient subgroups with different slopes of decline curves in order to find out in which patients the retardation effect is likely to be particularly marked.

TARGET SYMPTOMS OF A CHOLINERGIC TREATMENT

The question of target symptoms of cholinergic treatment of AD is important for three reasons:

- It is useful for determining the specificity of the cholinergic treatment for core symptoms of AD.

- It helps to understand the mode of action of cholinergic compounds.
- It may help to identify patient subgroups which are likely to profit most from a cholinergic treatment.

Preliminary analyses of the results obtained with velnacrine suggest that it has primarily the following cognitive effects:

- *Improvement of attentional functions* (Wesnes *et al.*, 1991: various vigilance tasks; the European phase II pilot study with velnacrine (202DZ): choice reaction time task; the European phase III enrichment study with velnacrine (301MN): digit symbol substitution task).
- *Improvement of recent (verbal) memory functions* (Wesnes *et al.*, 1991: test of word recognition and recall; Ebmeier *et al.*, 1992: word recognition; the European phase II pilot study with velnacrine (202DZ): word recognition; the European phase III enrichment study: paired-associate learning and carers' observations on NOSGER subscale 'Memory').

The above results describe only effects which were replicated in various studies using tests or scales with sufficient reliability and established validity to measure specific cognitive functions. Preliminary analyses of the ADAS cognitive subscale data suggest also effects on language and praxia functions (Siegfried, 1993b), but conclusions must be made with caution: single scale items are known to be less reliable than scale sum scores and well-constructed psychometric performance tests. Further more complex analyses are needed to reveal the whole spectrum of the cognitive effects of velnacrine and their relationship to effects on complex overlearnt habits and action sequences of everyday behavior. In this context it has to be pointed out that a clinical description of target symptoms is not the same as a causal analysis and interpretation of the compound's neuropsychological mode of action. The conclusion that the effects of cholinesterase inhibitors are due to a basic attentional effect (Sahakian and Coull, 1993) is a hypothesis which appears to have some validity but needs more scrutiny.

EFFECT SIZE AND FREQUENCY OF RESPONSE

The effect size of the aminoacridines has been a matter of controversial discussion on the clinical relevance of these drugs (Growdon, 1992). The discussion revolved around the magnitude of the *mean* verum–placebo difference on the ADAS cognitive subscale. In clinical trials with velnacrine, effect sizes were in a range of approximately 2 to 4.5 points, which is comparable to figures reported for tacrine. Although the effect size is an important factor in the determination of the statistical significance of effects, one has to be cautious to use it as a measure of the clinical relevance. The meaning of score differences is dependent on the scale type (e.g. rank scales, interval scales, absolute scales), the sensitivity, standard deviation, reliability, and standard error of measurement of the scale in question. Thus, a small score difference on one scale can represent a more relevant effect than a bigger one on another. Most important in the discussion of the clinical relevance of score differences is the external validity of the scale which is reflected in correlations with other measures (see the following section on clinical relevance).

Using the mean placebo–verum difference as an indicator of clinical relevance is also slightly misleading for another reason. Mean differences give a clinically inadequate impression of drug effects if there is a larger group of non-responders. In this case, a mean score difference represents a value in between those of responders and non-responders and is therefore representative for neither of the two groups. This is likely to occur when heterogeneous patient populations are investigated. In order to get a clinically more adequate impression of the relevance of the drug effects, it therefore appears to be necessary to determine the frequency of initial responders according to a predefined response criterion and find out for how long this effect is maintained. This response criterion must not only meet certain statistical prerequisites (i.e. the amount of change must exceed the standard error of measurement) but also have clinical validity. The criterion used in the velnacrine studies was an initial improvement of at least four points on the ADAS cognitive subscale. A four-point change does not only exceed the standard error of measurement (i.e. cannot be explained by mere chance), but also reflects a compensation of an approximately six-month deterioration of the disease and has also been shown to have biological correlates (Siegfried, 1993a).

CLINICAL RELEVANCE OF TREATMENT EFFECTS

The discussion of the clinical validity of effect sizes has emphasized the importance of adequate criteria for clinical relevance of treatment effects. The following criteria are suggested as valid indicators of clinical relevance:

- The relative frequency of drug responders must significantly exceed that of placebo responders. Such evidence will only be convincing if the response criterion has been predefined in the study protocol and meets the methodological prerequisites mentioned in the previous section.
- It must be demonstrated that the drug effects have an impact on patients' everyday behavior, most notably on functional habits in everyday life which help the patient to maintain a certain degree of independence (i.e. '(Instrumental) Activities of Daily Living') but also other areas of behavior which have an impact on patients' quality of life.
- Ideally, treatment should not only improve patients' behavior but also have an impact on patients' caregivers.
- Finally, the consistency of results of different measures obtained by separate observers is a convincing criterion of clinically relevance. Different measures and separate observers (e.g. comprehensive performance-based clinical observer rating scales; clinician's clinical global impression of change ratings; carer ratings of patients' everyday behavior; objective cognitive performance tests . . .) do not only pick up different aspects of the effects but also have different sensitivity thresholds. Therefore, consistency of results rules out that statistically significant effects could only be demonstrated due to the application of a highly sensitive measure which might assess changes that are practically irrelevant.

Most of the criteria for clinical relevance listed above have been suggested by the latest guidelines for the development of antidementia agents of the European Commission (CPMP, 1992). All of these criteria are met by the results obtained in clinical trials with velnacrine in patients with probable AD:

- Using the 4-point ADAS cognitive subscale change criterion, the responder rates varied between approximately 40 and 68% depending on the type of study and the assessment point used. In the dose-ranging segment of the phase II US velnacrine study, approximately 68% of patients showed a response and 42% of all patients had both acceptable safety results and response (Murphy *et al.*, 1991). After a three-week 'test treatment' with velnacrine, 68.3% of all treated patients of the European phase III enrichment study responded and 54.1% showed both a response and acceptable tolerance (Scheltens *et al.*, 1994). A life-table analysis (Kaplan and Meier, 1958) of response during the four-month double-blind placebo-controlled segment of the same study brought about the following cumulated responder frequencies: 54.9% in the velnacrine (50 mg t.i.d.) group as compared to 18.75% in the placebo group. The difference was highly significant (p = 0.008; Mantel-Cox or logrank test: see Greenhouse *et al.*, 1989). The velnacrine–placebo response frequency difference may even have been slightly underestimated in this trial due to carry-over effects from the test treatment phase.
- In both phase III trials, statistically significant differences in favor of velnacrine could be demonstrated on various measures of everyday behavior as rated by the patients' caregivers: after four months of treatment (endpoint) in the European study, there was a significant effect on the NOSGER subscales 'Memory' (p = 0.04) and 'Instrumental Activities of Daily Living' (p = 0.04). At baseline, these two subscales represented those two areas of everyday behavior where patients had most of their problems. Likewise, in the six-month US parallel-group trial, velnacrine proved to be statistically superior to placebo on the 'Physical Self-Maintenance Scale' (PSMS: Lawton and Brody, 1988) (p = 0.026) and the carers' global impression rating of patients' change (p = 0.005).
- In the latter study, a 'caregivers' allocation of time survey' (CATS) was used to estimate carers' time spent with the patient (for feeding, transporting, supervising, etc.) (Moore and

Clipp, 1994). Velnacrine (225 mg/day) was found to significantly reduce caregiver time requirements in comparison to placebo ($p \leq 0.03$). After six months of treatment, the time spent on care was reduced by 45% (3.2 hours per day) versus baseline ($p < 0.01$). The reduction in supervision time accounted for most of the differences because patients were able to live more independently.

- It has already been pointed out above (see section on evidence of efficacy above) that there was a consistency of the results obtained by separate observers (clinician, psychometrician, carers) on different scales (clinical global impression of change, ADAS cognitive subscale, cognitive performance tests, carers' ratings of everyday behavior; see also carers' time allocation survey).

THE RISK–BENEFIT RATIO

An ultimate judgement on the usefulness of the cholinergic treatment approach with aminoacridines like velnacrine must be based on a risk–benefit evaluation. This must take into consideration

- the risk and problems of untreated AD
- the benefits offered by a treatment, and
- the risk of a treatment attempt.

AD is a chronic illness with a high prevalence in elderly people. It is characterized by an inevitable downhill course which leads to complete loss of memory and intellectual functions and a decay of personality, and finally, approximately five to seven years after the first clinical diagnosis, results in the patient's death. This process involves a long and painful suffering of both the patient and his/her relatives, loads an enormous burden on the shoulders of the carers, and last but not the least causes huge health care costs for hospitalization and nursing home care in the later stages of the disease. So far no effective treatment for core signs and symptoms of the disease is available. Therefore the aminoacridines can be considered as first-generation AD agents. They offer an effective symptomatic treatment for a subgroup of patients and seem to retard the disease process for approximately one year. The treatment effects have an impact on patients' everyday behavior and are also likely to improve their caregivers' quality of life (reduction of supervision time; more time for themselves).

The risks of a treatment are:

- In approximately 20–30% (depending on the cut-off criterion used: twice or three times the upper limit of normal) of patients, significant increases in transaminase levels (SGPT, SGOT) occur. These are sometimes accompanied by increases of GGT, alkaline phosphatase, and LDH; but no significant increase of bilirubin has been observed. Patients are asymptomatic with the exception of mild asthenia in a few patients. Approximately 95% of all liver enzyme elevations occurred within a critical time window, namely between weeks four and twelve of treatment, and all values returned to normal upon discontinuation of the drug.
- The most frequent symptoms observed and reported in clinical trials with velnacrine as adverse events were peripheral cholinergic effects (gastric hypermotility such as diarrhea, nausea, vomiting). Each of these occurred in less than 10% of the patients. CNS symptoms (e.g. headaches, dizziness, agitation) represent the second category in the frequency of adverse events but comparisons of frequencies under verum and placebo suggest that these symptoms are likely to be a reflection of the underlying disease rather than true 'side-effects' of the drug.
- In rare cases, neutropenias were observed. These seem to occur within the same critical time window as liver enzyme elevations.

A risk–benefit evaluation comes to a favorable conclusion for the drug, provided certain precautions and prerequisites are observed: first, patients must undergo regular liver function and hematology tests. Secondly, patients' response should be evaluated early, i.e. after the first few weeks of treatment, and patients who do not seem to respond should be excluded. Since an efficacy evaluation can be made after approximately three to six weeks of treatment, non-responders can be excluded before liver enzyme elevations and—in rare cases—neutropenia are likely to occur. Thus the drug would be removed from patients who may have only a risk but no benefit.

LIMITATIONS OF A CHOLINERGIC TREATMENT APPROACH

Cholinesterase inhibitors of the class of aminoacridines (velnacrine, tacrine) are the first generation of effective AD agents. Although they seem to represent a major scientific and clinical advance, they clearly have their limitations, as could be expected from first-generation compounds:

- Only a subgroup of patients with the clinical diagnosis of 'probable AD' responds to this type of drug. This finding suggests that this diagnosis seems to cover a pharmacologically heterogeneous group. Non-responders may need a different treatment which may have to take into account a more complex neurotransmitter deficit. Unfortunately, there is not yet a biological or clinical marker which could help identify potential responders before drug exposure. This problem can be partly solved pragmatically through an initial test treatment. However, a real solution would require increased research activities to find variables that allow a clinically relevant subtyping of patients and prediction of response.
- Second-generation compounds would have to have an improved safety profile which, in particular, would make frequent laboratory tests unnecessary.
- A cholinergic treatment is no cure or causal therapy which could bring the disease process to an arrest. It can alleviate symptoms and at best slow down the disease process. It would therefore be desirable to have a causal treatment. However, etiological hypotheses of AD are still controversial among experts. It needs, for example, to be shown whether a drug which could stop amyloid accumulation in the development of senile plaques and neurofibrillary tangles would really bring the disease to an arrest. The usefulness of other types of neuroprotective mechanisms has also to be explored.

The attractiveness of the cholinergic deficit hypothesis of AD is the consistency of the supporting pathological and pharmacological evidence and the parsimony of its assumptions. The clinical results obtained with the aminoacridines in patients with AD demonstrate that it also has some clinical validity. However, the above-mentioned conclusion of a pharmacological heterogeneity of patients with 'probable AD' (according to NINCDS-ADRDA criteria) makes it obvious that further progress in treatment of AD needs an improved diagnostic classification system as well as reliable and valid tools for patient subtyping. This will not only help to improve symptomatic approaches but is a necessary prerequisite for finding a causative treatment.

REFERENCES

Agnoli, A., Martucci, N., Manna, V., Conti, L., and Fioravanti, R. (1983) Effect of cholinergic and anticholinergic drugs on short-term memory in Alzheimer's dementia: a neuropsychological computerised electroencephalographic study. *Clin. Neuropharmacol.*, **6**, 311–323.

Alzheimer, A. (1907) Über eine eigenartige Erkrankung der Hirnrinde. *Zentralblatt Neurol. Psychiat.*, **18**, 177–179.

Bartus, R. T., Dean, R. C., Pontecorvo, M. J., and Flicker, C. (1985) The cholinergic hypothesis: a historical review, current perspectives and future directions. *Ann. New York Acad. Sci.*, **444**, 332–358.

Beller, S. A., Overall, J. E., and Swann, A. C. (1985) Efficacy of oral physostigmine in primary degenerative dementia. A double-blind study of response to different dose levels. *Psychopharmacology*, **87**, 147–149.

Blackwood, D. H. R., and Christie, J. E. (1986) The effects of physostigmine on memory and auditory P300 in Alzheimer-type dementia. *Biol. Psychiatry*, **21**, 557–560.

Blennow, K. (1990) Heterogeneity of Alzheimer's disease. Doctoral Thesis from Department of Psychiatry and Neurochemistry. Univ. of Göteborg/Sweden.

Caltagirone, C., Gainotti, G., and Masullo, C. (1982) Oral administration of chronic physostigmine does not improve cognitive or mnestic performances in Alzheimer's presenile dementia. *Int. J. Neurosci.*, **16/3–4**, 247–249.

Christie, J. E., Phil, M., Shering, A., Ferguson, J., and Glen, A. M. (1981) Physostigmine and arecoline: effects of intravenous infusions in Alzheimer presenile dementia. *Br. J., Psychiatry*, **138**, 46–50.

CPMP (1992) CPMP working party on efficacy of medicinal products. Note for guidance. Antidementia medicinal products. Draft 5. Commission of the European Communities. Brussels.

Cohen, G. D. (1983) Historical views and evolution of concepts. In B. Reisberg (ed.), *Alzheimer's Disease.* The Free Press, New York, London, pp. 29–34.

Davidson, M., Mohs, R. C., and Hollander, E. (1986) Physostigmine in patients with Alzheimer's disease. *Psychopharmacol. Bull.*, **22/1**, 101–105.

Davies, P. (1981) Theoretical treatment possibilities for dementia of the Alzheimer type: the cholinergic hypothesis. In Th. Crook and S. Gershon (eds), *Strategies in the Development of an Effective Treatment for Senile Dementia.* Mark Powley, New Canaan, Connecticut, pp. 19–34.

Davis, K. L. and Mohs, R. C. (1982) Enhancement of memory processes in Alzheimer's disease with multiple-dose intravenous physostigmine. *Am. J. Psychiatry*, **139**, 1421–1424.

Davis, K. L., Mohs, R. C., Davis, B. M., Levy, M., Rosenberg, G. S., Horvath, T. B., De Nigris, Y., Ross, A., Decker, P., and Rothpearl, A. (1981) Cholinomimetic agents and human memory: Clinical studies in Alzheimer's disease and scopolamine dementia. In Th. Crook and S. Gershon (eds), *Strategies in the Development of an Effective Treatment for Senile Dementia.* Mark Powley, New Canaan, Connecticut, pp. 53–70.

Davis, K. L., Thal, L. J., Gamzu, E. R., Davis, C. S., Woolson, R. F., Gracon, S. F., Drachman, D. A., Schneider, L. S., Whitehouse, P. J., Hoover, T. M. *et al.* (1992) A double-blind, placebo-controlled multicenter study of tacrine for Alzheimer's disease. The Tacrine Collaborative Study Group. *N. Engl. J. Med.*, **327** (8), 1253–1259.

Drachman, D. A., and Leavitt, J. (1974) Human memory and the cholinergic system: a relationship of aging? *Arch. Neurol.*, **30**, 113–121.

Ebmeier, K. P., Hunter, R., Curran, S. M., Dougal, J., Murray, C. C., Wyper, D. J., Patterson, J., Hanson, M. T., Siegfried, K., and Goodwin, G. M. (1992) Effects of a single dose of acetylcholinesterase inhibitor velnacrine on recognition memory and cerebral blood flow in Alzheimer's disease. *Psychopharmacology*, **108**, 103–109.

Fielding, S., Cornfeldt, M. L., Szewczak, M. R., Ellis, D. B., Huger, F. P., Davis, K. L., Wilker, J. C. and Shutske, G. M. (1989) HP029, a new drug for the treatment of Alzheimer's disease: its pharmacological profile. In H. Kewitz, T. Thomson, and U. Bickel (eds), *Pharmacological Interventions on Central Cholinergic Mechanisms in Senile Dementia (Alzheimer's Disease).* W. Zuckschwerdt Verlag, München, Bern, Wien, San Francisco.

Folstein, M. F., Folstein, S. F., and McHugh, P. R. (1975) Mini-mental state: a practical method for grading the cognitive state for the clinician. *J. Psychiatr. Res.*, **12**, 189–198.

Gottfries, C. G. (1989) Alzheimer's disease—one, two or several. *J. Neural Transm. (Parkinson's Disease and Dementia Section)*, **1**, 22.

Gottfries, C. G. (1993) Classification of Alzheimer type dementia. In E. C. Wolters and Ph. Scheltens (eds), *Alzheimer's Disease: Back to the Future*. Vrije Universiteit Amsterdam, pp. 21–27.

Greenhouse, J. B., Stangel, D., and Bromber, J. (1989) An introduction to survival analysis: statistical methods of clinical trial data. *J. Consult. Clin. Psychol.*, **57**, 533–544.

Growdon, J. H. (1992) Treatment for Alzheimer's disease? *N. Engl. J. Med.*, **327** (18), 1306–1308.

Haefner, H. (1989) Epidemiology of dementia. *J. Neural Transm. (P–D Section)*, **1**, 3.

Hoff, P., and Hippius, H. (1989) Alois Alzheimer 1864–1915. Ein Überblick über Leben und Werk anlässlich seines 125. Geburtstags. *Nervenarzt*, **60**, 332–327.

Holford, N. H., and Peace, K. E. (1992) Results and validation of a population pharmacodynamic model for cognitive effects in Alzheimer patients treated with tacrine. *Proc. Natl Acad. Sci. USA*, **89** (23), 11471–11475.

Inglis, J. (1959) A paired-associate learning test for use with elderly psychiatric patients. *J. Ment. Sci.*, **105**, 440–443.

Kaplan, E. L., and Meier, P. (1958) Nonparametric estimation for incomplete observations. *J. Am. Statist. Assoc.*, **53**, 457–481.

Lawton, M. P., and Brody, E. M. (1988) Physical Self-Maintenance Scale (PSMS): original observer-rated version. *Psychopharmacol. Bull.*, **24**, 793–795.

McKhann, G., Drachman, D., Folstein, M., Katzman, R., Price, D., and Stadlan, E. M. (1984) Clinical diagnosis of Alzheimer's disease: Report of the NINCDS-ADRDA work group under the auspices of the department of health and human services task force on Alzheimer's disease. *Neurology*, **34**, 939–944.

Moore, M. J., and Clipp, E. C. (1994) Alzheimer's disease and caregiver time. Letter to editor. *Lancet*, **343**, no. 8891.

Murphy, M. F., Hardiman, St., Nash, R. J., Huff, F. J., Demkovitch, J. J., Dobson, C., and Knappe, U. F. (1991) Evaluation of HP029 (velnacrine maleate) in Alzheimer's disease. *Ann. NY Acad. Sci.*, **640**, 253–262.

National Institute of Mental Health (NIMH) (1976) Clinical Global Impressions. In W. Guy (ed), *ECDEO Assessment Manual for Psychopharmacology*. Rev. Ed. Rockville, Maryland, 217–222.

Perry, E. K. (1987) Cortical neurotransmitter chemistry in Alzheimer's disease. In H. Y. Meltzer (ed.), *Psychopharmacology. The Third Generation of Progress.* Raven Press, New York, pp. 887–896.

Perry, E. K., Gibson, P. H., Blessed, G., Perry, R. H., and Tomlinson, B. E. (1977) Neurotransmitter enzyme abnormalities in senile dementia. Choline acetyltransferase and glutamic and decarboxylase activities in necropsy brain tissue. *J. Neurosci.*, **34**, 247–265.

Perry, E. K., Tomlinson, B. E., Blessed, G., Bergman, K., Gibson, P. H., and Perry, R. H. (1978) Correlation of cholinergic abnormalities with senile plaques and mental test scores in senile dementia. *Br. Med. J.*, **ii**, 1457–1459.

Puri, S. K., Hsu, R., Ho, I., and Lassman, H. B. (1988) Single-dose safety, tolerance, and pharmacokinetics of HP029 in elderly men: a potential Alzheimer's agent. *Curr. Ther. Res.*, **44**, 766–780.

Rosen, W., Mohs, R., Davis, K. (1984) A new rating scale for Alzheimer's disease. *Am. J. Psychiatry*, **141**, 1356–1364.

Rosen, W. G., Terry, R. D., Fuld, P. A., Katzman, R., and Peck, A. (1980) Pathological verification of ischemic score in differentiation of dementias. *Ann. Neurol.*, **7**, 486–488.

Sahakian, B. J., and Coull, J. T. (1993) Tetrahydroaminoacridine (THA) in Alzheimer's disease: an assessment of attentional and mnemonic function using CANTAB. *Acta Neurol. Scand.* (Supplement) **149**, 29–34.

Scheltens, Ph., Siegfried, K., Dartigues, J. F., De Deyn, P., Derouesne, C., Horn, R. *et al.* (1994) The effects of velnacrine in the treatment of patients with mild to moderately severe degrees of Alzheimer's disease—Results of a European multicentre trial. Submitted for publication.

Siegfried, K. (1992) Der heuristische Wert der Hypothese eines zentralen cholinergen Defizits beim Morbus Alzheimer als Ausgangspunkt einer pharmakologischen Behandlungsstrategie. In J. Oldigs-Kerber and J. P. Leonard (eds), *Pharmakopsychologie.* Gustav Fischer Verlag, Jena, Stuttgart, pp. 459–470.

Siegfried, K. (1993a) The pharmacodynamics of velnacrine: results and conclusions from clinical studies in healthy subjects and patients with Alzheimer's disease. In G. K. Wilcock (ed.), *The Management of Alzheimer's Disease.* Wrightson Biomedical Publishing Ltd., Petersfield, UK, pp. 189–202.

Siegfried, K. (1993b) Pharmacodynamic and early clinical studies with velnacrine. *Acta Neurol Scand.* (Supplement) **149**, 26–28.

Siegfried, K., and Murphy, M. F. (1993) The cholinergic approach to the treatment of Alzheimer's disease. In E. Ch. Wolters and Ph. Scheltens (eds), *Alzheimer's Disease. Back to the Future.* Vrije Universiteit, Amsterdam, pp. 97–106.

Spiegel, R. (1989) The NOSGER (Nurses' Observation Scale for Geriatric Patients). August 1989 (distributed by the author).

Wechsler, D. (1958) *The Measurement and Appraisal of Adult Intelligence.* Williams & Wilkins, Baltimore.

Wesnes, K. (1985) A fully automated psychometric test battery for human psychopharmacology. Fourth World Congress of Biological Psychiatry, Philadelphia, September (Abstracts).

Wesnes, K., Simpson, P., White, L., Pinker, S., Murphy, M., and Siegfried, K. (1991) Cholinesterase inhibition in the scopolamine model of dementia. *Ann. NY Acad. Sci.*, **640**, 268–271.

Wilcock, G. K. (1991) Scientific basis for therapeutic developments in Alzheimer's disease. In I. Hindmarch, H. Hippius, and G. K. Wilcock (eds), *Dementia. Molecules, Methods and Measures.* John Wiley & Sons, Chichester, New York, Brisbane, Toronto, pp. 61–66.

Wilkins, R. H., and Brody, I. A. (1969) Alzheimer's disease. *Arch. Neurol.*, **21**, 109–110.

5

Gangliosides Selectively Diminished in Early-onset Alzheimer's Disease (AD Type I) Suggest Synapse Loss as Primary Event

L. Svennerholm, C. G. Gottfries, and I. Karlsson

University of Göteborg, Department of Clinical Neuroscience, Mölndal, Sweden

ABSTRACT

Brains from 12 cases of Alzheimer's disease early onset (AD type I) and 21 cases of senile dementia of Alzheimer type (type II) were investigated. Frontal gray matter, temporal gray matter, the caudate nucleus and hippocampus and white matter tissue from the frontal lobe were carefully dissected. Gangliosides, phospholipids, cholesterol, cerebroside and sulfatide were determined. AD type I had significantly lower concentrations of gangliosides in all areas when compared to those in the AD type II group and age-matched controls. In AD type II significant reduced ganglioside concentrations were found in the temporal lobe and in the hippocampus only as compared with the age-

Alzheimer's Disease: Clinical and Treatment Perspectives. Edited by N. R. Cutler, C. G. Gottfries and K. Siegfried.

matched controls. Phospholipids were significantly reduced in all gray matter areas in the type I group when compared to age-matched controls and the type II group. Membrane lipids in white matter showed an opposite turn. Significantly reduced concentrations were recorded for phospholipids, cholesterol, cerebroside and sulfatide in the type II group when compared to age-matched controls and the type I group. The data indicate fundamental biochemical differences in the two major forms of Alzheimer-type dementia. In the type I group there is a loss of gangliosides, indicating a reduction in neuronal processes, whereas loss of myelin lipids is the major characteristic of the type II form. The findings suggest that the two forms of Alzheimer-type dementia do not have the same pathogenesis.

INTRODUCTION

Originally, Alzheimer's disease (AD) was characterized as a presenile dementia with neuropathological hallmarks of senile plaques and neurofibrillary tangles. In the 1970s, senile dementia of nonvascular type was renamed senile dementia of the Alzheimer type (SDAT) and sampled with AD, because it was assumed that both disorders were of the same type and that differences in symptoms were due to differences in age at onset. At present, however, there is a body of evidence suggesting that Alzheimer-type dementia is a heterogeneous group of disorders (for review see Blennow, 1990).

In the presenile form, the symptoms have onset before the age of 65. However, thorough clinical investigations have shown that, in the presenile form (AD type I), a parieto-temporal symptomatology dominates which is not found in SDAT (type II). Moreover, nonregional symptoms, such as memory impairment and impairment of abstract thinking, problem solving ability, and logical/analytical ability, dominate in type II but not in type I. In type II the presence of delirium states is significantly more frequent than in the type I form (Blennow *et al.*, 1990). Brain imaging data also appear to differentiate the two forms. In type II there is white matter degeneration in 91% of cases, whereas white matter degeneration is found in only 33% in type I (Blennow *et al.*, 1991). As is evident from Blennow *et al.* (this volume, Chapter 2), cerebrospinal fluid (CSF) and neurochemical data also indicate differences between the two forms. Increased concentrations of gangliosides and decreased concentrations of chromogranin A are found in type I as compared with type II. Taken together, these clinical data indicate that type I is a gray matter disorder in which the damage to the parieto-temporal lobes appears to dominate. The neurochemical findings may also suggest a loss of synapses. Postmortem findings of imipramin and GBR-12935-binding to brain tissue (putamen) of Alzheimer-afflicted patients also indicate a loss of serotonergic and dopaminergic synapses in AD/SDAT (Marcusson *et al.*, 1987; Allard *et al.*, 1990).

Ganglioside loss and loss of membrane components have been reported by several investigators (Suzuki *et al.*, 1965; Bowen *et al.*, 1973, 1977, 1979; Bowen and Davison, 1986; DeKosky and Bass, 1982; Sorbi *et al.*, 1987; Nitsch *et al.*, 1992; Kienzl *et al.*, 1993). The findings are not concise, but usually they are interpreted as showing a neuronal loss or a selective axodendritic degeneration. In our own studies gangliosides were reduced in the caudate nucleus and the reduction was more evident in patients with early onset than in those with late onset (Gottfries *et al.*, 1983).

The aim of the present study was to investigate membrane components in well-defined type I and type II cases and compare them with age-matched controls. The data are presented in more detail in Svennerholm and Gottfries (1994).

MATERIAL AND METHODS

The group of AD type I included 12 cases, 7 females and 5 males with a duration of disease of 5.7 ± 2.5 years, and 21 cases of AD type II, 11 females and 10 males with a duration of disease of 5.5 ± 2.8 years. The diagnosis was made as described by Blennow *et al.* (1990, 1991). In the autopsy room 20 subjects, 10 females and 10 males with durations of agonal stages similar to those of the demented subjects, were selected as controls.

Macroscopic Examination of the Brain

Excluding cases with vascular brain diseases and other pathological changes not concomitant with the diagnosis of AD/

SDAT, microscopic examination confirmed the diagnoses of AD/SDAT.

The frontal gray matter (Brodmann 9) and temporal gray matter (Brodmann 21–22) were carefully peeled off and deep-frozen at –80 °C. The caudate nucleus and hippocampus were carefully dissected, while surrounding white matter tissue was avoided, and then deep-frozen. White matter from the frontal lobe was dissected. The frozen samples were pulverized with a powder homogenate from which the lipids were extracted for neurochemical investigations. Gangliosides expressed as μmoles lipid-bound sialic acid were determined together with phospholipids, cholesterol, cerebroside, and sulfatide. For methods see Svennerholm and Gottfries (1994).

Statistics

Significance analyses for group comparisons of quantitative parameters were performed using the Wilcoxon two-sample test.

RESULTS

As is evident from Table 1 and Figure 1, gangliosides in gray matter were significantly reduced in all four areas investigated when AD type I was compared with age-matched controls. In type II differences were found in the temporal lobe and in the hippocampus. When AD type I was compared with type II, there were significantly lower concentrations in the AD type I group in all areas investigated. Phospholipids were significantly reduced in all gray matter areas investigated when AD type I was compared with age-matched controls. No reduced concentrations were found in gray matter of patients with the type II form. When AD type I was compared with type II, reduced concentrations were found in the former in the frontal lobe, temporal lobe, caudate nucleus, and hippocampus (Table 1, Figure 2). Cholesterol was significantly reduced in the caudate nucleus and hippocampus in AD type I when compared with age-matched controls.

Table 1 *Major membrane lipids of four gray matter areas of Alzheimer brains*

	Controls 1	AD type I	Controls 2	AD type II	Significance levels AD II vs AD I
Frontal lobe	$n = 16$	$n = 11$	$n = 12$	$n = 21$	
Phospholipids (μmol/g)	38.3 ± 4.0	33.5 ± 2.1****	36.7 ± 3.6	36.7 ± 2.9	$p<0.01$
Cholesterol (μmol/g)	23.0 ± 2.1	21.0 ± 2.1	21.6 ± 2.0	21.2 ± 2.1	n.s.
Gangliosides (μmol/g)	2.92 ± 0.30	2.02 ± 0.35****	2.80 ± 0.23	2.70 ± 0.28	$p<0.0001$
Temporal lobe	$n = 13$	$n = 11$	$n = 12$	$n = 18$	
Phospholipids (μmol/g)	41.4 ± 7.7	33.8 ± 3.2**	38.1 ± 5.2	36.1 ± 3.8	n.s.
Cholesterol (μmol/g)	24.9 ± 4.3	21.5 ± 2.7	23.1 ± 3.0	20.7 ± 2.1	n.s.
Gangliosides (μmol/g)	3.30 ± 0.47	1.91 ± 0.42****	3.10 ± 0.33	2.68 ± 0.38**	$p<0.001$
Caudate nucleus	$n = 16$	$n = 11$	$n = 12$	$n = 21$	
Phospholipids (μmol/g)	48.1 ± 3.2	38.6 ± 5.0***	45.9 ± 3.8	43.6 ± 4.6	$p<0.05$
Cholesterol (μmol/g)	33.4 ± 6.1	28.5 ± 5.1*	31.2 ± 4.9	28.1 ± 3.9	n.s.
Gangliosides (μmol/g)	3.03 ± 0.34	1.92 ± 0.27****	2.83 ± 0.24	2.80 ± 0.35	$p<0.0001$
Hippocampus	$n = 15$	$n = 12$	$n = 13$	$n = 20$	
Phospholipids (μmol/g)	47.0 ± 5.3	35.0 ± 5.8****	42.9 ± 4.6	41.5 ± 6.4	$p<0.05$
Cholesterol (μmol/g)	38.2 ± 5.4	25.7 ± 6.5***	32.1 ± 5.0	31.6 ± 7.0	n.s.
Gangliosides (μmol/g)	2.42 ± 0.40	1.61 ± 0.30****	2.17 ± 0.34	1.93 ± 0.21*	$p<0.01$

Ganglioside values are expressed in μmoles of lipid-NeuAc.
* $p< 0.05$, ** $p<0.01$, *** $p<0.001$, **** $p<0.0001$.

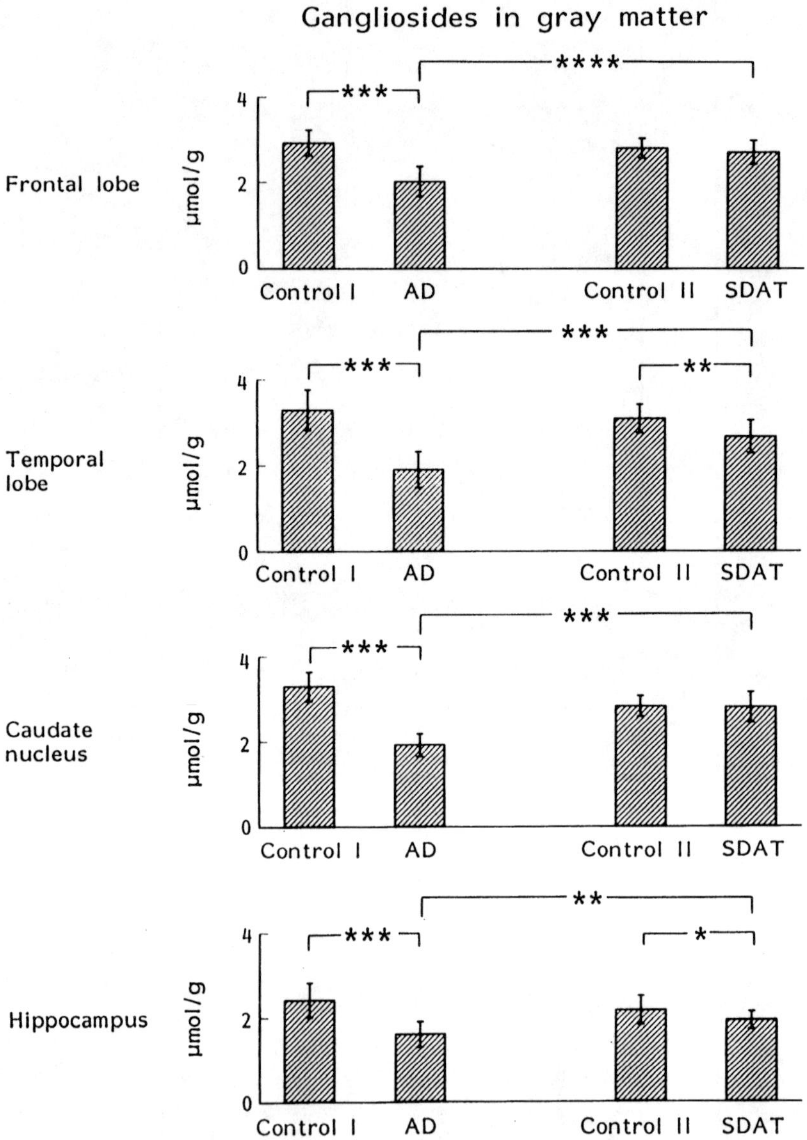

Figure 1 *Differences in concentrations of gangliosides in age-matched controls I (n = 13–16), Alzheimer's disease with early onset (AD; age at onset < 65; n = 11–12), age-matched controls II (n 12–13), and senile dementia of the Alzheimer type (SDAT; age at onset p ≥ 65; n = 20–21). ** p < 0.01, *** p < 0.001, **** p < 0.0001*

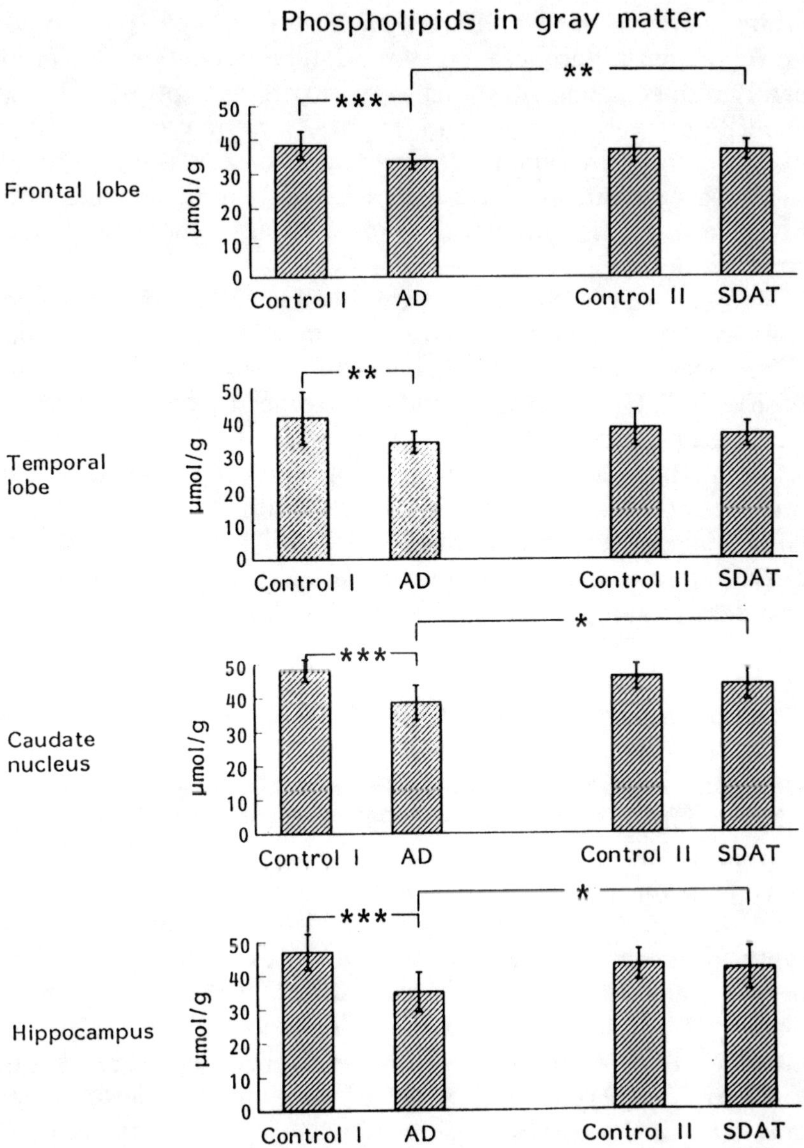

Figure 2 *Differences in concentrations of phosphiolipids in age-matched controls I* (n = *13–16), Alzheimer's disease with early onset (AD; age at onset* < *65;* n = *11–12), age-matched controls II* (n *12–13), and senile dementia of the Alzheimer type (SDAT; age at onset* ≥ *65;* n = *20–21).* * p < *0.05,* ** p < *0.01,* *** p < *0.001*

As is evident from Table 2 and Figure 3, membrane lipids in white matter showed a different pattern of damage. In AD type I no significant differences were found, whereas in type II, significantly reduced concentrations were recorded for phospholipids, cholesterol, cerebroside, and sulfatide compared with age-matched controls. When AD type I was compared with type II, there were significant differences with more reduced concentrations in type II concerning phospholipids, cholesterol, and cerebroside.

Significant differences in the ganglioside pattern between controls and AD cases were only seen in AD type I. The major differences from the controls consisted in an increase in ganglioside GD3, GM2 and GM1 and a decrease in the proportions of GD1a and GT1b in the four gray areas and also in the frontal white matter. The increase in the proportion of GD3 is probably due to reactive astrocytosis, while the diminution of GD1a and GDT1b suggests an inhibition of sialyl transferase IV, the enzyme that catalyzes the transfer of sialic acid to the terminal galactose of gangliosides of the gangliotetraose series.

DISCUSSION

The concentration of gangliosides—marker for axodendritic arborization—was reduced to 58–70% of the control concentration in all four gray areas ($p<0.0001$) and to 81% of the control concentration in the frontal white matter ($p<0.01$) of AD type I cases. In type II cases the ganglioside concentration was significantly reduced only in the temporal cortex, hippocampus and frontal white matter and to a lesser extent, 86%, 87% and 94%, respectively. The concentration of phospholipids was also significantly reduced in all four gray areas of AD type I cases, but in no area of AD type II cases. The diminution of cholesterol was only 50% of the corresponding phospholipid reduction in AD type I cases. These results suggest a pronounced loss of nerve endings in AD type I, which was confirmed by the demonstration of a diminished yield in the isolation of synaptosomes from the affected gray areas.

The characteristic membrane lipid disturbance in AD type II was a loss of myelin lipids in the frontal white matter:

Table 2 *Major membrane lipids of frontal white matter of Alzheimer brains*

	Controls 1	AD type I	Controls 2	AD type II	Significance levels AD II vs AD I
	n = 12	*n* = 10	*n* = 10	*n* = 18	
Phospholipids (μmol/g)	98.4 ± 7.3	91.3 ± 13.3	93.1 ± 12.2	79.0 ± 12.8**	p<0.05
Cholesterol (μmol/g)	116.9 ± 14.4	112.2 ± 17.0	105.0 ± 12.9	90.6 ± 17.3*	p<0.001
Cerebroside (μmol/g)	39.7 ± 5.7	41.5 ± 7.2	39.3 ± 5.9	31.7 ± 6.6***	p<0.001
Sulfatide (μmol/g)	16.6 ± 3.8		16.0 ± 4.3	10.2 ± 2.1**	
Gangliosides (μmol/g)	1.18 ± 0.14	0.96 ± 0.13**	1.08 ± 0.12	1.01 ± 0.12*	n.s.

Ganglioside values are expressed in μmoles of lipid-NeuAc.
* p< 0.05, ** p<0.01, *** p<0.001.

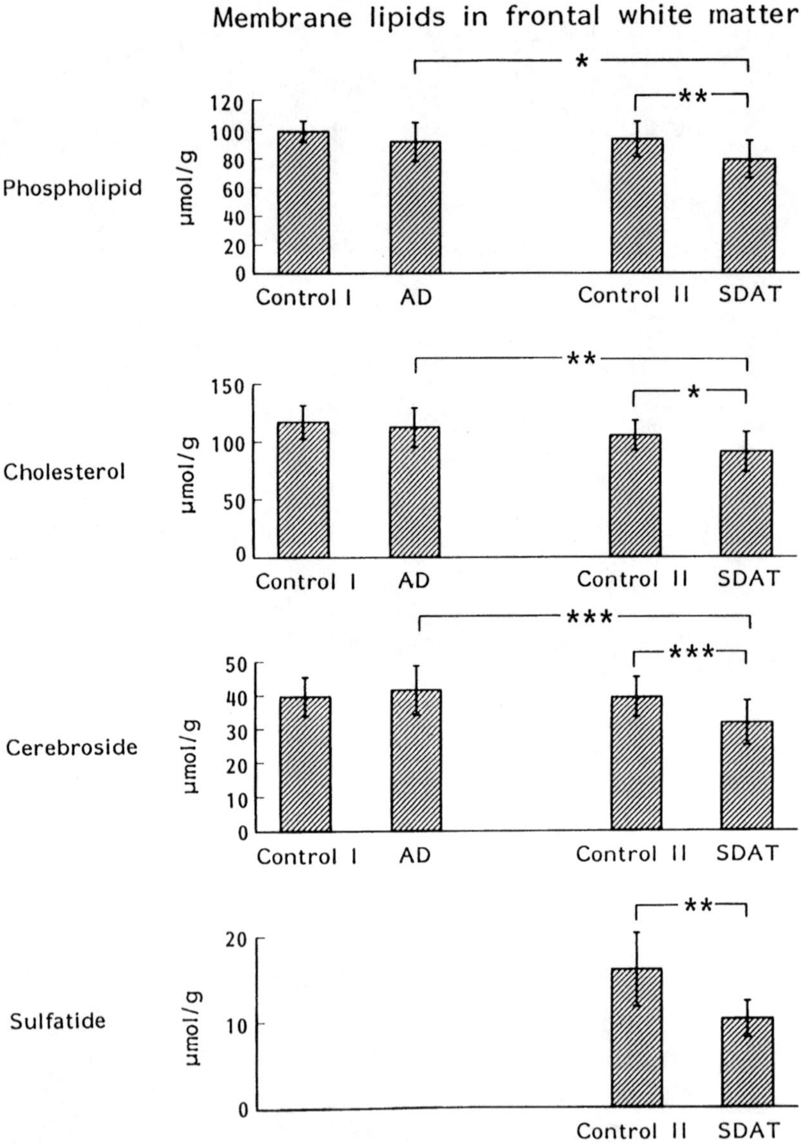

Figure 3 *Concentrations of membrane lipids in frontal white matter in age-matched controls I* (n = 12)*, Alzheimer's disease with early onset (AD; age at onset < 65;* n = *10), age-matched controls II* (n = *10), and senile dementia of the Alzheimer type (SDAT; age at onset ≥ 65;* n = *18).* * p < *0.05,* ** p < *0.01,* *** p < *0.001*

cerebroside, cholesterol, phospholipids, and sulfatide, while no significant loss of myelin lipids was recorded in AD type I. This is the first time a fundamental biochemical difference has been shown between two major forms of Alzheimer-type dementia—a generalized loss of gangliosides as a sign of profound reduction in neuronal processes in AD type I and a loss of myelin lipids as a sign of demyelination in SDAT type II. These findings demonstrate that the two forms of AD do not have the same pathogenesis.

Our study of membrane lipids in AD type I showed a pronounced loss of the lipids that form the cellular processes, particularly the synapses, while the neuronal cell bodies and the axons appear to be relatively well preserved. It would then be possible to stimulate the outgrowth of the nerve endings. Gangliosides have been shown to possess neurotogenic and neuronotrophic properties (Ledeen, 1984). Therefore, we began to administer GM1 ganglioside subcutaneously to patients with AD type I. However, pharmacokinetic studies revealed that gangliosides do not penetrate an intact blood–brain barrier (BBB; Svennerholm *et al.*, 1990). For this reason, we began to administer GM1 intraventricularly. Shunt catheters are implanted into the frontal part of the lateral ventricles and are connected to a Rickham reservoir, which will allow sampling of cerebrospinal fluid during the treatment. A fine teflon catheter is connected to a micropump that will continuously infuse GM1 solution into the ventricles. Five patients have been treated with GM1 for more than one year. So far there have been no adverse effects of the treatment. The patients are assessed with a battery of psychological tests and rating scales. No dramatic effect has been recorded, but some variables have improved. As the study is open, so far no valid conclusions can be drawn. The aim is to operate on a total of ten patients.

ACKNOWLEDGEMENTS

This research was supported by grants from the Swedish Medical Research Council (B93-21X-05002); the Fidia Research Laboratories, Abano Terme, Italy; the Bank of Sweden Tercentenary Foundation (861–326); Stridhs Fond and Ödmans Fond,

Göteborgs Läkaresällskap; Barbro Hanssons och Göteborgs Kvinnliga Handlares Fonder; Stiftelsen Söderström-Königska Sjukhemmet; Forsknings- och Utvecklingsfonden; Gun och Bertil Stohnes Stiftelse; Konung Gustaf V:s och Drottning Victorias Stiftelse; Torsten och Ragnar Söderbergs Stiftelser; Fredrik and Ingrid Thurings Stiftelse; Stiftelsen Gamla Tjänarinnor; and Lundbeckfonden.

REFERENCES

Allard, T., Alafuzoff, I., Carlsson, A., Eriksson, K., Ericson, E., Gottfries, C. G., and Marcusson, J. O. (1990) Loss of dopamine uptake sites labeled with (^{3}H)GBR-12935 in Alzheimer's disease. *Eur. Neurol.*, **30**, 181–185.

Blennow, K. (1990) Heterogeneity of Alzheimer's disease. Doctoral Thesis. Medical Faculty of the University of Göteborg, Sweden.

Blennow, K., Wallin, A., and Gottfries, C. G. (1990) Confusional symptomatology distinguishes early- and late-onset Alzheimer's disease. *Aging*, **2**, 395–401.

Blennow, K., Wallin, A., Uhlemann, C., and Gottfries, C. G. (1991) White matter lesions in Alzheimer's disease—relation to clinical symptomatology and vascular factors. *Acta Neurol. Scand.*, **83**, 187–193.

Bowen, D. M., and Davison, A. N. (1986) Biochemical studies of nerve cells and energy metabolism in Alzheimer's disease. *Br. Med. Bull.*, **42**, 75–80.

Bowen, D.M., Smith, C. B., and Davison, A. N. (1973) Molecular changes in senile dementia. *Brain*, **96**, 849–856.

Bowen, D. M., Smith, C. B., White, P., Flack, R. H. A., Carrasco, L. H., Gedye, J. L., and Davison, A. N. (1977) Chemical pathology of the organic dementias II. Quantitative estimation of cellular changes in post-mortem brains. *Brain*, **100**, 427–453.

Bowen, D. M., Spillane, J. A., Curzon, G., Meier-Ruge, W., White, P., Goodhardt, M. J., Iwangoff, P., and Davison, A. N. (1979) Accelerated ageing or selective neuronal loss as an important cause of dementia? *Lancet*, **i**, 11–14.

DeKosky, S. T., and Bass, N. H. (1982) Aging, senile dementia and the intralaminar microchemistry of cerebral cortex. *Neurology*, **32**, 1227–1233.

Gottfries, C. G., Adolfsson, R., Aquilonius, S. M., Carlsson, A., Eckernäs, S. Å., Nordberg, A., Oreland, L., Svennerholm, L., Wiberg,

Å., and Winblad, B. (1983) Biochemical changes in dementia disorders of Alzheimer type (AD/SDAT). *Neurobiol. Aging*, **4**, 261–271.

Kienzl, E., Puchinger, L., Jellinger, K., Stachelberger, H., and Varmuza, K. (1993) Studies of phospholipid composition in Alzheimer's disease brain. *Neurodegeneration*, **2**, 101–109.

Ledeen, R. W. (1984) Biology of gangliosides: neuritogenic and neuronotrophic properties. *J. Neurosci. Res.*, **12**, 147–159.

Marcusson, J. O., Alafuzoff, I., Bäckström, I. T., Ericson, E., Gottfries, C. G., and Winblad, B. (1987) 5-Hydroxytryptamine-sensitive (^{3}H)imipramine binding of protein nature in the human brain. II. Effect of normal aging and dementia disorders. *Brain Res.*, **425**, 137–145.

Nitsch, R. M., Blusztajn, J. K., Pittas, A. G., Slack, B. E., Growdon, J. H., and Wurtman, R. J. (1992) Evidence for a membrane defect in Alzheimer's disease brain. *Proc. Natl Acad. Sci. USA*, **89**, 1671–1675.

Sorbi, S., Piacentini, S., and Amaducci, L. (1987) Intralaminar distribution of neurotransmitter-related enzymes in cerebral cortex of Alzheimer's disease. *Gerontology*, **33**, 197–202.

Suzuki, K., Katzman, R., and Korey, S. R. (1965) Chemical studies in Alzheimer's disease. *J. Neuropathol. Exp. Neurol.*, **22**, 629–642.

Svennerholm, L., and Gottfries, C. G. (1994) Membrane lipids selectively diminished in Alzheimer brains suggest synapse loss as primary event in early onset form (Type I) and demyelination in late onset form (Type II). *J. Neurochem.*, **62**, 1039–1047.

Svennerholm, L., Gottfries, C. G., Blennow, K., Fredman, P., Karlsson, I., Månsson, J. E., Toffano, G., and Wallin, A. (1990) Parenteral administration of GM1 ganglioside to presenile Alzheimer patients. *Acta Neurol. Scand.*, **81**, 48–53.

6

Alzheimer's Disease: Is the Improvement of Cholinergic Transmission the Correct Strategy?

D. M. Bowen[1], P. T. Francis[1], I. P. Chessell[1], M-T. Webster[1], A. W. Procter[1,2], C. P. L-H. Chen[1,3], M. Qume[1], D. Neary[4], A. J. Cross[5], and A. R. Green[5]

[1]Miriam Marks Department of Neurochemistry, Institute of Neurology, Queen Square, London, UK. [2] Department of Psychiatry, United Medical and Dental School (Guy's Campus), London, UK. [3]Department of Neuropathology, Radcliffe Infirmary, Oxford, UK. [4]Department of Neurology, Manchester Royal Infirmary, Manchester, UK. [5]Astra Neuroscience Research Unit, London, UK

ABSTRACT

An effective neurotransmitter-related drug that may improve the clinical response rates found with tacrine could probably be developed. It should have the properties of both a cholinomimetic (either a acetylcholine esterase inhibitor or muscarinic m_1 receptor agonist) and a serotonin 1A receptor antagonist. Such a drug should also beneficially affect the digestion of amyloid precursor

Alzheimer's Disease: Clinical and Treatment Perspectives. Edited by N. R. Cutler, C. G. Gottfries and K. Siegfried.

protein by the brain. These conclusions are based on features of degenerative dementias which include the selective degeneration of subpopulations of corticocortical glutamatergic pyramidal neurons and maintained (or increased) inhibitory tone (features of Alzheimer's and Pick's diseases, also of dementia of frontal lobe type) as well as the presynaptic cholinergic deficit (Alzheimer and Lewy body dementias). In combination, these features are considered to cause hypoactivity of other glutamatergic pyramidal neurons involved in cognition in these dementias. The variable response to tacrine is probably related to structural changes that co-exist as well as too few patients in some clinical trials. In conclusion, to further drug development it is important to persevere to improve activity of the remaining circuits of glutamatergic neurons.

INTRODUCTION

Some ten years after the introduction in 1968 of L-dopa therapy for Parkinson's disease, a substantial presynaptic cholinergic abnormality in the brains of patients with Alzheimer's disease (AD) suggested a basis for rational pharmacological treatments. An additional effect of such neurotransmitter replacement is now emerging as processing pathways for β-amyloid precursor protein (APP) appear to be regulated by transmitter receptors, at least those coupled to the phosphoinositide (PI)/Ca^{2+} second messenger system such as the acetylcholine muscarinic (m_1) receptor (Nitsch *et al.*, 1992). Figure 1 shows that activation of this receptor favors the non-amyloidogenic pathway (α-secretase) that leads to a decrease in the intracellular amyloidogenic fragments generated from APP (Fukushima *et al.*, 1993). There is controversy regarding the mechanism by which mismetabolism of APP might cause cell death as it is not certain that β-amyloid protein is toxic in AD brain. Moreover, although harmful alterations in energy metabolism in AD have been hypothesized by several authorities, the evidence that this is capable of contributing to either mismetabolism of APP or toxicity of the amyloid protein remains far from definitive (Francis *et al.*, 1993b). There is evidence, however, that should an oxidative stress be a pathogenic factor then transmitter therapy would be useful if aimed at the PI/Ca^{2+} system (Table 1; Figure 1).

Table 1 *Effect of neurotransmitter-related agents and an oxidative stress on secretion of APP derivatives from a human-like cell line (nerve growth factor-differentiated PC12 cells)*

Agent added, normal or stressed cells	APP derivative	
	KPI	695
None		
normal	100	100
stressed	68 ± 7 (7)	65 + 8 (7)*
Bradykinin (500 nM)		
normal	165 ± 15 (10)*	187 ± 15 (10)*
stressed	94 ± 17 (3)	89 ± 27 (3)
Phorbol ester (100 nM)		
normal	151 ± 17 (4)	161 ± 9 (4)*
stressed	101 ± 18 (3)	91 ± 16 (3)
Nicotine (10 μM)		
normal	123	105
Nicotine (100 μM)		
normal	101	98
Nicotine (1 mM)		
normal	79	99
Lithium (1.5 mM)	149 ± 22 (4)	151 ± 17* (4)

Mean ± SEM (n, number of independent experiments) of APP in medium as percent of value for normal cells without agent added (nicotine values are mean of two experiments showing similar trends).

* Significantly different from control, *t* statistic. Oxidative stress was induced by the addition of oligomycin and deoxyglucose in glucose-free medium (adenosine triphosphate was decreased by 50%). APPs (approx. 110–140 kDa) were detected with commercial antibody 22C11, an antibody to aa 1–16 of β-amyloid protein (Dr D. Allsop) and antibody 7H5 which recognizes the KPI domain (Dr D. Schenk) (Webster *et al.*, 1993, M-T. Webster, P.T. Francis, and D.M. Bowen, unpublished observations).

Postmortem biochemical studies of AD, where extensive transmitter deficits may be seen, have led some workers to the pessimistic conclusion that a transmitter-based therapy cannot be successful. However, such studies almost invariably examine the end-stage of this slowly progressing disease and this is rarely acknowledged in the interpretation. It has been possible to study samples removed earlier in the disease as neocortical tissues from AD patients have been occasionally removed surgically for diagnostic purposes. Transmitter changes in neurosurgical (biopsy) samples, and the comparison of these with the corresponding evidence obtained from postmortem studies, have been emphasized in this chapter.

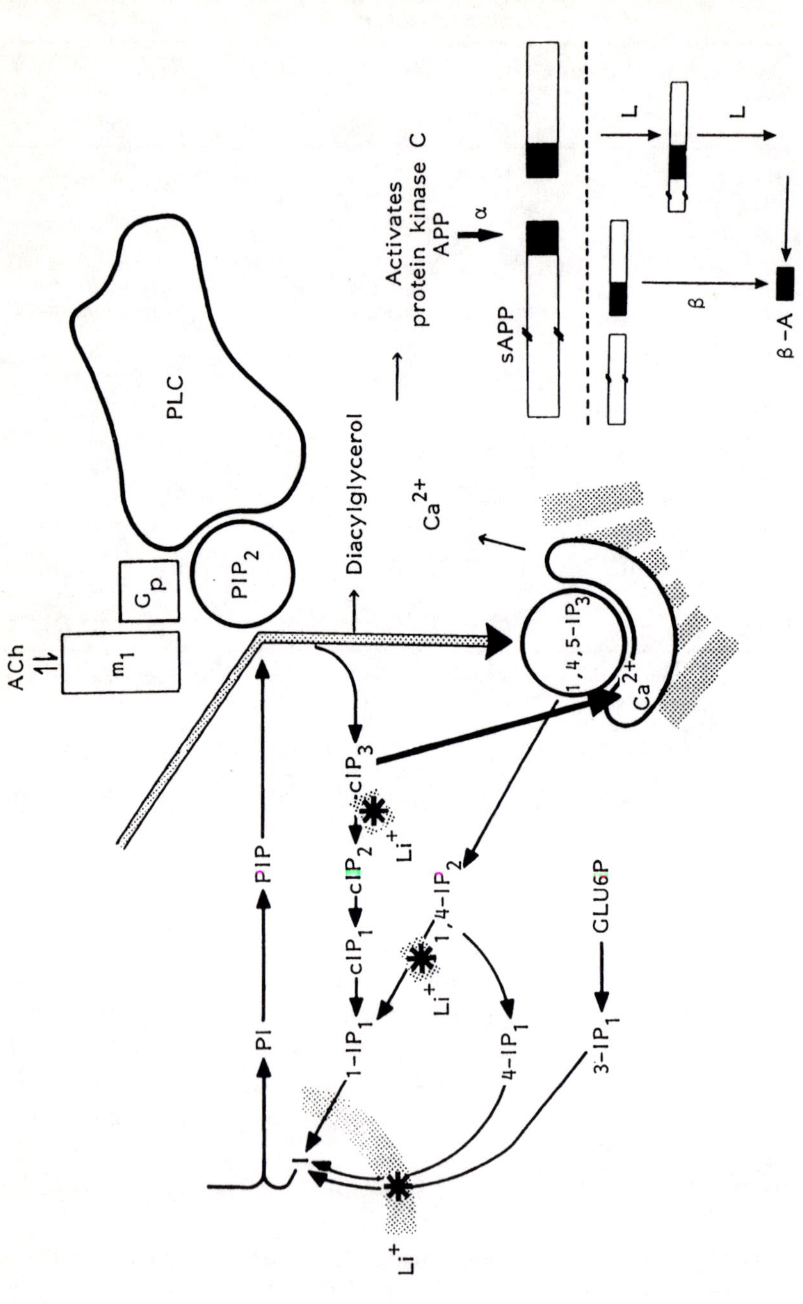
ACh
m_1
G_p
PIP_2
PLC
Diacylglycerol
Activates protein kinase C
APP
α
sAPP
L
L
β
β-A
Ca^{2+}
1,4,5-IP_3
Ca^{2+}
cIP_3
Li^+
cIP_2
cIP_1
PI
PIP
1-IP_1
Li^+
1,4-IP_2
4-IP_1
GLU6P
3-IP_1
Li^+

SUBCORTICAL NEUROTRANSMITTERS

Transmitter systems in the region of the cell bodies of cholinergic nucleus basalis neurons may provide approaches for ameliorating cholinergic dysfunction in AD (as reviewed, Francis *et al.*, 1992a; 1993b). An interesting recent observation was that although 5-hydroxyindole acetic acid (5-HIAA) and serotonin (5-HT) concentrations were reduced their ratio, an index of 5-HT turnover, was increased (Sparks *et al.*, 1992).

CORTICOPETAL NEUROTRANSMITTERS

By contrast with cholinergic inputs in the brain of AD patients, those using the catecholamines, noradrenaline and dopamine, are relatively unaffected. The situation regarding inputs using 5-HT is complex. Even in autopsy AD brain, half of the many cortical areas assayed showed no evidence of a selective reduction in presynaptic 5-HT activity. Hence, deficiency of presynaptic serotonergic activity is probably never widespread, a feature consistent with the preservation of 5-HIAA concentration in ventricular CSF (VCSF) from living AD patients. Indeed, the turnover rate in those 5-HT nerve endings remaining appears to be enhanced in AD patients, based on the increased ratio of 5-HIAA to 5-HT in cortical tissue and the nucleus basalis. Furthermore, 5-HIAA concentration in lumbar CSF was positively

Figure 1 *Diagrammatic summary of the effect of acetylcholine (ACh) on signal transduction in a pyramidal neuron (Figure 2) membrane (Figure 3) muscarinic m_1 receptor coupled to phospholipase C (PLC) and phosphoinositide (PI) turnover and showing the relationship to the effects of Li^+ (Agranoff, 1989; Stubbs and Agranoff, 1993; Berridge, 1993) and the metabolism of APP (text). In this model, secretion of APP derivatives from PC12 cells (Table 1) was increased by acute (1 hour) exposure to Li^+, presumably due to the accumulation of IP_3 (breakdown inhibited by Li^+, asterisk) releasing calcium from the endoplasmic reticulum to stimulate APP metabolism by the α-secretase pathway (α), involving activation of protein kinase C. Chronic Li^+ administration in combination with antidepressants (Table 5) inhibited PI recycling (indicated by asterisks), so according to this model and in sequence: phosphatidylinositol bisphosphate (PIP_2) and diacylglycerol concentration were decreased; APP metabolism by α-secretase was inhibited; β-secretase pathway (β) and/or lysomal processing (L) were favored; β-amyloid protein (β-A) accumulated; efflux of APP derivatives was decreased so VCSF values were reduced*

correlated with dementia rating in a series of histologically verified living AD patients, and in another series the mean 5-HIAA value was significantly higher than control (Francis *et al.*, 1994). Recently we have found that for AD subjects dying in the community the concentrations of 5-HT and 5-HIAA were not significantly reduced in the areas studied (frontal and temporal cortex). Indeed, in the temporal cortex the ratio of 5-HIAA to 5-HT was increased (p=0.004, for log transformed data, Student's t test) in AD (22.8 ± 14.1 units, n = 19) compared to controls (13.8 ± 4.8 units, n = 12; J. T. Alder, C. Chen, P. T. Francis and D. M. Bowen, unpublished observations). This extends earlier work as long-stay psychiatric hospitals were the probable source of almost all previously studied autopsy material and these are likely to represent a skewed population due to the inadvertent selection of subjects with non-cognitive behavioral problems. Dementia of frontal lobe type (DFT) and Pick's disease, characterized by some of these behaviors, are similar to AD as there is evidence of increased 5-HT turnover (Francis *et al.*, 1993a, 1993b) but there is no observed cholinergic hypoactivity (Francis *et al.* 1993a; Table 2). DFT is considered to be part of a clinical syndrome which includes Pick's disease, another disorder that does not seem to be characterized by cholinergic hypoactivity (Table 2). It could be argued, therefore, that it is important to exclude such patients from clinical trials of cholinomimetic agents. This is not the case with senile dementia of

Table 2 *Chemical pathology of the superior frontal cortex in various dementias*

Diagnosis	ChAT activity (pmol ACh/ mg protein/min)	m_1 Binding (fmol/mg protein)	Somatostatin (fmol/mg protein)
Control (26)	97 ± 56	9.5 ± 4.5	146 ± 76
AD (9)	47 ± 26*	9.1 ± 3.0	155 ± 104
DFT (6)	94 ± 42	8.9 ± 4.4	254 ± 86*
DFT with MND (5)	124 ± 36	8.6 ± 4.7	165 ± 61
MND (6)	92 ± 25	9.1 ± 5.4	135 ± 56
Pick's disease (10)	90 ± 45	7.4 ± 3.4	207 ± 80*

Mean ± SD (n). * indicates statistically different from control, $p < 0.05$, ANOVA followed by multiple comparison test. ChAT and MND identifies choline acetyltransferase and motor neuron disease respectively; DFT with MND and Pick's disease are less common than DFT (Mann *et al.*, 1993; Neary *et al.*, 1993); M. Qume and A.J. Cross, unpublished observations.

the Lewy body type (as described by Perry *et al.* (1990); see also Hansen *et al.* (1990) who considered this to be only a variant of AD) where choline acetyltransferase activity was severely reduced.

Neurosurgical samples showed a severe deficiency in acetylcholine synthesis by the mid-point of AD, detailed clinical assessments of these patients have been made, and the rating of dementia was correlated with synthesis, but showed no correlation with the transmitters of the other corticopetal neurons. Sparing of catecholamines was confirmed (as reviewed, Francis *et al.*, 1992a).

CORTICAL INHIBITORY NEUROTRANSMITTERS AND NEUROPEPTIDES

The balance of evidence indicates that GABA, glycine, taurine, cholecystokinin, vasoactive intestinal polypeptide, neuropeptide Y and somatostatin are not critically depleted in AD. It is well known that somatostatin content provides a useful index of a category of GABA interneurons. Preservation of these would indicate maintained inhibitory tone on cortical pyramidal neurons (Figure 2) and this appears to be a feature of DFT and Pick's disease (Table 2).

HIPPOCAMPAL NEUROTRANSMITTERS

In the hippocampus all the major input and output pathways (except the septohippocampal cholinergic pathway) use L-glutamate (GLU) as transmitter (Figure 2). There was cell loss and tangle formation in the entorhinal cortex and in CA1 in AD patients at postmortem. Indeed, *in vivo* imaging suggests that atrophy of the hippocampus occurs by the mid-point of the disease process (Kesslak *et al.*, 1991). GLU concentration postmortem in the terminal zone of the perforant pathway was decreased by 80% in AD specimens. Consistent with this, decreased GLU staining was observed in the molecular layer of the dentate gyrus. It was noted that GLU and glutaminase immunoreactive pyramidal neurons in the CA fields were decreased in number and the remaining neurons showed irregular

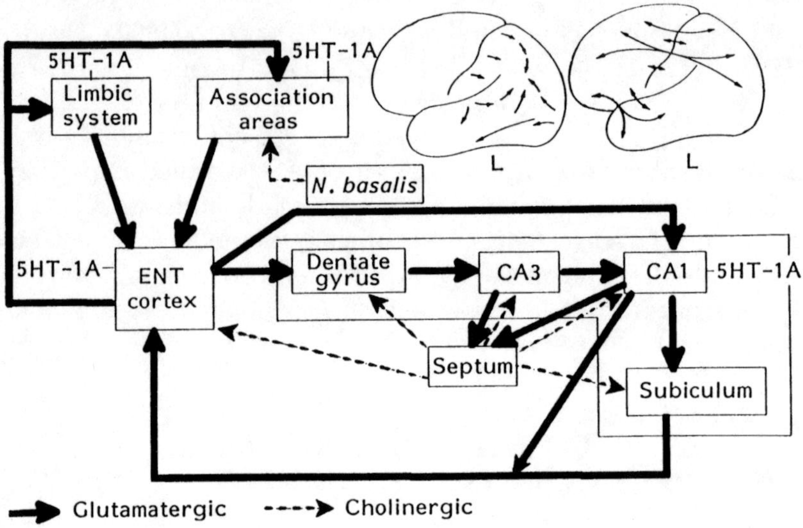

Figure 2 *Diagrammatic representation of glutamatergic pyramidal neuron pathways of the brain thought to underlie cognitive processes. ENT, identifies entorhinal cortex. Limbic system, identifies components other than the hippocampus and ENT (e.g. cingulate cortex). Large box identifies hippocampus. Relationships are also shown between glutamatergic pathways and cholinergic innervation from the septum and the nucleus basalis. Some cortical association pathways are shown for the lateral surface of the brain (L). 5-HT*$_{1A}$ *receptors are probably enriched on pyramidal neurons in the areas indicated. Brain region distribution determinations indicate that ENT, dentate gyrus and association pathways have many 5-HT*$_{1A}$ *receptors. These, along with muscarinic m*$_1$ *receptors, help to regulate cortical glutamatergic pyramidal neurons (Figure 3)*

shortening and disorganized dendritic fields. Many also showed tangle formation (as reviewed, Kowall and Beal, 1991). Thus if the GLU pathways are considered to be involved in memory it follows that the loss of GLU function may contribute to the memory dysfunction in AD. Loss of ChAT activity together with reduced synaptosomal choline uptake indicated that major presynaptic cholinergic pathology was also a feature of the hippocampus in AD (as reviewed, Francis *et al.*, 1993b).

EXCITATORY NEOCORTICAL NEUROTRANSMITTERS

Three studies indicated that severity of dementia correlated with degeneration of corticocortical pyramidal neurons in association areas (Neary *et al.*, 1986; DeKosky and Scheff, 1990; Terry *et al.*, 1991). Although there are difficulties in separating transmitter GLU from the large metabolic pools, a combination of techniques has provided evidence for a transmitter role for GLU in a number of pathways, including corticortical pyramidal neurons. The temporal and parietal lobes of AD patients may be major and early sites of pathological changes, as these regions showed reductions in glucose metabolism as assessed by positron emission tomography, a measurement in living brain which is sensitive to atrophy. Psychological test scores correlated with both the positron emission tomography data, and pyramidal cell counts in cortical layer III and number of synapses in layer III. Thus, a clinically relevant shrinkage or loss of association fibers probably occurred from circumscribed (i.e. parietotemporal) areas and this contributed to the overall reduction observed in glucose metabolism.

In summary, there is now evidence accumulating that GLU is the principal transmitter of the corticortical association fibers and the major hippocampal pathways (Figure 2). Histological and scanning studies indicate that these pathways degenerate quite early in AD and some neurochemical data support this (as reviewed, Francis *et al.*, 1992a, 1993b).

CORTICAL NEUROTRANSMITTER RECEPTOR SYSTEMS

Studies on postmortem AD samples have indicated that binding sites for most transmitters are unaltered in the cerebral cortex (as reviewed, Francis *et al.*, 1992a). The main postsynaptic muscarinic receptor (m_1) seemed to be preserved (Table 2), which should provide a suitable target for acetylcholine. Nicotinic and m_2 muscarinic receptors (at least the latter may be primarily presynaptic) were reduced. Binding sites for 5-HT were not consistently abnormal. Altered populations of binding sites for GLU have been reported in the hippocampus but little change was seen in the neocortex, although reduced GLU binding in cortical layers I and II has been reported. Apart from reduced sensitivity to modulation by glycine, the properties of the NMDA receptor complex seem to be normal but the number of complexes may be reduced, probably due to pyramidal cell loss (Steele *et al.*, 1992). Penney and colleagues used quantitative receptor autoradiography to measure m_1, benzodiazepine and various GLU binding sites in sections of the hippocampal region. The binding loss was greater for NMDA sites than for m_1. Jansen and colleagues also found reduced NMDA receptors. By contrast, [^{3}H]kainate binding was not reduced (and even increased in the neocortex), as was found by Chalmers, Dewar and colleagues. Quisqualate-dependent GLU binding estimates two subtypes of receptor; one of these, the α-amino-3-hydroxy-5-methyl-4-isoxazolepropanoic acid site, was reduced (as reviewed, Francis *et al.*, 1992a). The other site, the metabotropic receptor (but see Schoepp and True (1992), where subtypes are discussed), was also reduced. 5-HT$_2$ receptors were reduced whereas the 5-HT$_1$ subtypes have not been studied (Francis *et al.*, 1992a).

Harrison and Pearson have established reliable *in situ* hybridization methods using ^{35}S-labelled oligonucleotides for the detection and quantification of the cell type capable of producing a given receptor. In two of the most affected cortical areas the mRNA for the m_1 receptor was increased whereas that for one of the receptor's probable G proteins was not affected. Although the amounts of cortical 'G protein' are reported to remain unchanged (see Francis *et al.*, 1992a) evidence has been presented indicating alterations in the functional integrity of some G proteins. This has been studied carefully by Cowburn and colleagues (Cowburn *et al.*, 1992), albeit at the endpoint of the disease (i.e. in autopsy samples). Changes also occur in the cerebellum, a region not showing hallmark histological lesions. Moreover, 5-HT$_{1A}$ receptor–G protein interactions were preserved in AD patients as was found for the m_1 receptor by Pearce and Potter (but not by Flynn and colleagues). However, the groups studying m_1 did not consider factors such as patients' immediate preterminal state (as reviewed, Pearce and Potter, 1991; Francis *et al.*, 1992a).

RECEPTOR REGULATION OF CORTICAL PYRAMIDAL NEURONS

Background

The regional and laminar distribution of receptors (including many subtypes) in the cerebral cortex are well known, yet the cellular localization of many is not clearly understood. The excitability of pyramidal neurons of the neocortex is affected by many transmitters, based on *in vitro* electrophysiological studies (as reviewed, McCormick and Williamson, 1989). However, such studies have consistently shown that only a proportion of cells respond to a particular drug, which suggests that there is a substantial degree of heterogeneity with respect to the transmitter receptors on pyramidal neurons.

It is well established that volkensin, a retrogradely transported toxic lectin from the kilyambiti plant, can be used to selectively destroy subpopulations of cortical and hippocampal pyramidal neurons distant from the site of injection (for a review see, Wiley, 1992). By this mechanism, unilateral intrastriatal volkensin injections lead to loss of large, infragranular, pyramidal neurons of the rat frontal cortex with preservation of glutamic acid decarboxylase (GAD) mRNA-positive interneurons (Pangalos *et al.*, 1991). Francis and colleagues (Pangalos *et al.*, 1991, 1992; Francis *et al.*, 1992b) have used receptor autoradiography with sections of rat brain from volkensin-injected animals to establish whether the affected subpopulation of cortical pyramidal cells (layer V corticostriatal projection neurons, a category of corticofugal neuron) are enriched with a particular receptor type. Corticocortical and corticofugal pyramidal neurons are probably subject to qualitatively similar regulation, irrespective of species (McCormick and Williamson, 1989), so it is hoped that the approach will provide better understanding of the transmitter receptor regulation of cortical pyramidal neurons in general.

These studies may have particular relevance for treatment and the improved diagnosis of neurodegenerative disorders such as AD, where loss of cortical pyramidal neurons underlies the pathology of the condition. This is because some receptors may provide the basis for development of novel ligands for *in vivo* brain imaging (as reviewed, Francis *et al.*, 1993a, 1993b; Chessell *et al.*, 1993) as well as targets for drug therapy. The substantial presynaptic cholinergic abnormality, accompanied by adequate coupling of the appropriate receptor (muscarinic m_1) in the brains of AD patients has been described above and this has suggested the basis of a rational palliative treatment (e.g. acetylcholinesterase inhibition).

In volkensin-treated animals we have previously reported on only one receptor that uses phosphatidylinositol bisphosphate PIP_2 hydrolysis (Figure 1), the 5-HT_2 receptor. A further study extends the receptors investigated to other phospholipase C (PLC, Figure 1) -linked receptors, m_1 and adrenoceptors (α_{1total} and the subtype α_{1b}). We have used [^{3}H]pirenzepine to label muscarinic receptors (predominantly the m_1 subtype, Buckley and Burnstock, 1986; Hulme *et al.*, 1990) and [^{3}H]prazosin to label α_1 receptors (α_{1total}), and in the presence of 5-methyl urapadil to label the α_{1b} subtype (Zilles *et al.*, 1991). The research has also been extended to the localization of m_1 receptors on corticocortical neurons.

Results

Intrastriatal injection of volkensin produced a significant loss of infragranular pyramidal neurons with preservation of GAD mRNA positive interneurons (Chessell *et al.*, 1994). This was also a feature of intracortical injections where a subpopulation of contralateral transcallosally projecting (a category of corticortical) pyramidal neurons was selectively destroyed. Table 3 summarizes the results for receptor localization based on the changes in volkensin-injected rats.

Implications

The study has emphasized the importance of m_1 receptors for regulating the activity of both corticofugal and corticocortical pyramidal neurons. This is based on the small but *consistent* reductions in binding of [^{3}H]pirenzipine to m_1 receptors in areas of neocortex that showed pyramidal neuron loss. From this work the most selective marker of the subpopulation of cor-

Table 3 *Summary of receptor localization*

Receptor	Pyramidal neurons		
	Corticofugal area		Corticocortical
	Medial	Lateral	
$5\text{-}HT_{1A}$	++	++	—
m_1	+	±	+
Nicotine	++	±	+
Kainate	+	—	nd
NMDA	+	—	nd
$GABA_A$	—	—	nd
$5\text{-}HT_2$	—	—	—
Adenosine A_1	—	—	—
$\alpha_{1\ total}$	—	—	nd
α_{1b}	—	—	nd

++, obvious enrichment; +, enriched; ±, some evidence of enrichment; —, no enrichment; nd, not determined (Chessell *et al.*, 1994).

ticofugal neurons is the $5\text{-}HT_{1A}$ receptor. Although this does not appear to be true for corticortical neurons in the rat, an important species difference should be emphasized. In rats $5\text{-}HT_{1A}$ receptors are found in the lower cortical layers whilst in primates (including man) there is an additional high density in upper layers. This observation suggests that the receptor is enriched on ipsilateral projecting corticocortical pyramidal neurons (Francis *et al.*, 1993b). Receptors that are present in the greatest numbers are obvious targets for drugs to normalize activity of these neurons. The most suitable receptors by other criteria are those that are PLC-linked (Figure 1) and may avoid the possibility of excitotoxicity. *Hence, positive modulation of impulse flow by the* m_1 *receptor, perhaps in combination with an antagonist of the* $5\text{-}HT_{1A}$ *receptor induced hyperpolarization, is considered to represent a most promising therapeutic strategy* (Figure 3). A further approach suggested by others (Court and Perry, 1991) is the use of nicotinic agonists. This is supported by the present study as these receptors appear to be enriched on pyramidal neurons (Table 3). Acetylcholinesterase inhibitors are well known to be under development for the treatment of AD and these should stimulate both nicotinic and m_1 receptors. However, our results indicate that nicotine has no obvious effect on APP secretion (Table 1), although the cells investigated possess nicotinic receptors (Madhok, 1993).

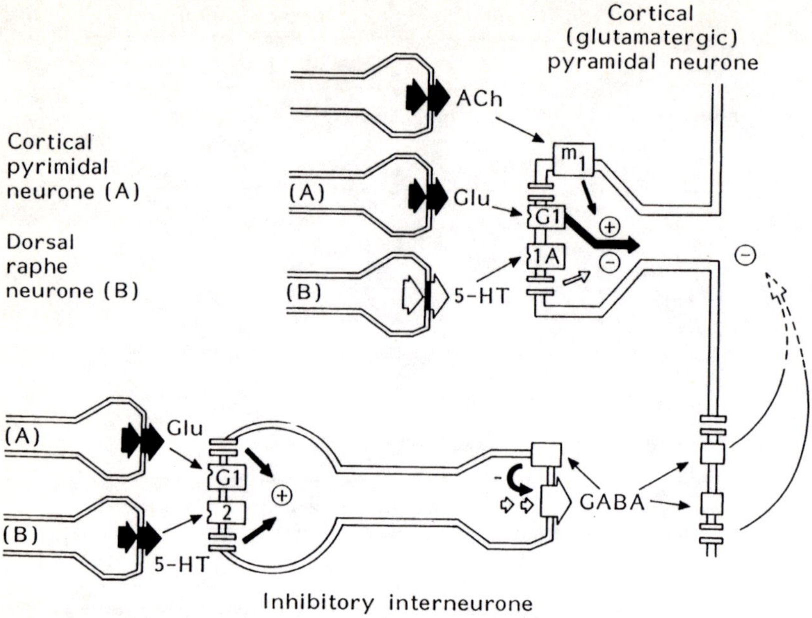

Figure 3 *Diagrammatic representation of the effects of transmitter receptors in a pyramidal neuron membrane on glutamatergic activity. In AD these neurons characteristically contain tangles and are lost, leading to reduced excitatory input (GLU) into the remaining neurons. This appears to be compounded by reduced excitatory cholinergic modulation (ACh). There is evidence that GABA neurons are preserved and this suggests that inhibitory tone is maintained, or perhaps increased. Other evidence (text) suggests functional sparing of serotonergic innervation and hence a negative modulatory effect via $5\text{-}HT_{1A}$ receptors. Direct acting GLU agonists have been viewed with caution as a therapy for AD because of the risk of excitotoxic damage. However, approaches which improve the efficacy of the remaining GLU transmission may be useful. Examples of how this may be achieved are shown—receptor agonists (via muscarinic, m_1 receptors) and antagonists (via $5\text{-}HT_{1A}$ receptors); as well as improving impaired cognition these should favor non-pathogenic cleavage of APP, via α-secretase (Figure 1)*

Our model (Figure 3) may provide clues for treatment strategies for non-Alzheimer dementias, exemplified here by DFT and Pick's disease. Although there is no obvious presynaptic cholinergic deficit, inhibition of acetylcholinesterase may compensate for the increased inhibitory tone mediated by 5-HT and interneurons. *Thus, a therapeutic strategy aimed at cholinergic transmission will probably be useful for DFT and Pick's disease as well as AD and senile dementia of the Lewy body type.*

AMYLOID PRECURSOR PROTEIN AND CORTICAL PYRAMIDAL NEURONS

Background

It is now recognized that in AD, neuronal loss from the frontal and temporal association cortex (Figure 2) is primarily a disappearance of glutamatergic pyramidal neurons, greater degeneration being associated with higher dementia scores (as reviewed, Neary *et al.*, 1986; Terry *et al.*, 1991; Francis *et al.*, 1993b). Of the two regions, the temporal cortex is the most degenerate. The remaining pyramidal neurons of cortical layer III are among the most obvious sites of neurofibrillary tangle formation (Braak and Braak, 1985; Pearson *et al.*, 1985; Lewis *et al.* 1987). Cortical pyramidal neurons in general appear to contain much of the APP found in the brain (as reviewed, Shigematsu *et al.*, 1992). Glial cells in culture have also been shown to express APP but do not appear to secrete large amounts of the protein (as reviewed, Haass *et al.*, 1991). It is well known that APP is subject to rare, dementia-producing, genetic mutations and this has been interpreted as the strongest evidence that the common non-familial form of AD results from APP mismetabolism leading to deposition of β-amyloid protein. Tau and apolipoprotein E, both found associated with tangles, bind to β-amyloid with high avidity (as reviewed, Poulter *et al.*, 1993; Saunders *et al.*, 1993), and this, together with mismetabolism of APP, is thought to be involved in the pathogenic events underlying sporadic AD. APP metabolism may be regulated by neuronal activity, in particular transmitter transduction mechanisms. This includes m_1 receptors, present on pyramidal neurons, which use products of PIP_2 hydrolysis as second messengers and, following activation, increase APP secretion by the α-secretase pathway (Figure 1; see also Nitsch *et al.*, 1992, 1993; Buxbaum *et al.*, 1992; Sinha and Lieberburg, 1992).

We have attempted to link the data for receptor enrichment on pyramidal neurons with results for APP in human brain to advance a hypothesis regarding pyramidal neurons, APP and the treatment of AD. This approach has been facilitated by using postmortem brain tissue from AD patients and controls collected specially using techniques designed to minimize autolysis (Procter *et al.*,

1990). Concentrations of the major species of APP have been determined in a soluble fraction and two membrane fractions from the cerebral cortex. We have also investigated any intercorrelations of these measures with numbers of pyramidal neurons and astrocytes as well as with a putative biochemical index of interneurons (γ-aminobutyric acid, GABA, content).

Results

Immunoblots with the APP antibody 22C11 revealed the same 4 bands of high apparent molecular mass 90–160 kDa (Webster *et al.*, 1994) as previously described in human cerebral cortex by various authorities. Antibody 22C11 has been used for quantification but samples have also been examined with other antibodies not generally available in order to define further the protein species present. The band in the soluble fraction with the characteristics of APP containing the Kunitz protease inhibitory (KPI) domain (APP_{KPI}) correlated with the number of pyramidal neurons, but not other cellular markers, in cerebral cortex (Francis *et al.*, 1993c). The correlation was observed with both antibody 22C11 and 10D5 (epitope mapped to β-amyloid protein 1–16, Chessell *et al.*, 1994). The study has also identified an APP_{695}-like soluble protein(s) which was higher in concentration in the brain of patients with AD compared with those from controls (patients with other dementias, Table 4).

Implications

It is doubtful whether any meaningful results would have been obtained had the study not employed the specially obtained postmortem tissue. Conclusions can be drawn with confidence because potentially confounding factors have been controlled for or investigated. This rigorous standard for comparison makes it virtually impossible to obtain brains of normal subjects matched to AD cases for these factors so the group of other dementias represent a more appropriate control (Procter *et al.*, 1990), albeit composed of several quite different disease entities (Webster *et al.*, 1994). The study provides evidence that secretion of APP from pyramidal neurons may be regulated by the state of receptor activation, since APP_{KPI} correlated inversely with the number of pyramidal neurons (i.e. the APP content was highest in tissue with the least neurons) and APP_{695} was increased in AD. Hence, a putative accumulation of APP within remaining pyramidal neurons has been linked to reduced receptor activation consequent upon degeneration of other pyramidal neurons (Francis *et al.*, 1993c). Almost certainly this would be exacerbated in AD by loss of excitatory cholinergic modulation (Figure 3; Francis *et al.*, 1993b; Chessell *et al.*, 1993).

AMYLOID PRECURSOR PROTEIN-LIKE IMMUNOREACTIVITY CAN BE ALTERED IN HUMANS BY DRUGS AFFECTING NEUROTRANSMITTER FUNCTION

Background

There are no drugs presently in routine clinical use which would be expected to *increase* APP secretion, in contrast to those used in studies of the cultured cell lines. Yet in affective disorders, lithium is prescribed and our *a priori* hypothesis was that since it is considered to interfere with PIP_2 recycling (Figure 1), such chronic treatment would be associated with lower APP concentrations in VCSF. APP secretion may also be decreased by drugs with anticholinergic or other neuronal activity inhibiting properties such as antidepressants. Therefore, we have examined the effect of therapy with these and other drugs, on indices of APP secretion in rare samples of human VCSF (Clarke *et al.*, 1993). The samples were obtained during perioperative air encephalography from patients undergoing stereotaxic psychosurgery for intractable depression. Drug treatments received in the two weeks prior to the operation were recorded and classified into five categories: antipsychotics, other tranquillizers, lithium salts, other antidepressants, and other drugs. On the basis of the *a priori* hypothesis (above) patients were divided into four groups according to treatment with lithium or antidepressants (Table 5).

Table 4 *APP-like immunoreactivity in neocortical fractions isolated from two categories of patients with clinical dementia*

Fraction	Frontal cortex		Temporal cortex	
	AD	Others	AD	Others
Soluble				
Band 2 (APP_{KPI})	1262 ± 170	1284 ± 294	1758 ± 95[a]	1626 ± 66[b]
Band 3 (APP_{695})	2282 ± 248	1889 ± 244	2398 ± 64[a,g]	2066 ± 65[b]
Band 4 (APP_{695})	403 ± 88[f]	127 ± 62	597 ± 68[a,d]	412 ± 66[b]
High density membranes				
Band 1 (APP_{KPI})	436 ± 45	465 ± 51	385 ± 44[a]	497 ± 44[b]
Band 2 (APPH)	808 ± 102	862 ± 79	750 ± 32[a]	851 ± 43[b]
Band 3 (APP_{695})	297 ± 65	349 ± 39	574 ± 14[a,e]	631 ± 29[b]
Low density membranes				
Band 1[c] (?)	253 ± 38[a]	238 ± 40[b]	151 ± 24[a]	103 ± 20[b]
Band 2[c] (?)	561 ± 65[a]	514 ± 53[b]	661 ± 64[a,d]	529 ± 37[b]
Band 3[c] (?)	203 ± 30[a]	194 ± 35[b]	293 ± 40[a]	264 ± 36[b]

Arbitrary units/mg protein, are mean ± SEM for 14 and 8 AD and other diagnosis patients, respectively, except where given ([a] 9–10 subjects [b] 6 sujects). Total protein contents of equivalent fractions from AD and other cases were not significantly different (data not shown). ( ) identifies probable major species (or derivative). Superscript [c] identifies bands affected by epiphenomena based on GAD activity and influence of terminal coma. Superscripts [d–g] identify the only differences between AD values and the equivalent values of the other patients ([d] $p < 0.1$, [e] $p < 0.05$, [f] $p < 0.02$, [g] $p < 0.01$, Mann-Whitney *U*-test) (Webster *et al.*, 1994).

Table 5 *Drug effects on antibody 22C11 immunoreactive species in VCSF*

Drug treatment	*n*	APP-like immunoreactivity (units)	
		KPI	695
Control	15	33 ± 7	18 ± 3
Antidepressant	25	23 ± 6	13 ± 2
Lithium	7	24 ± 6	11 ± 2
Lithium and antidepressant	38	16 ± 3*	10 ± 1

Values are mean ± SEM. Units are arbitrary units/mg total protein. * Mean significantly different from control (patients not receiving lithium or antidepressant but a drug from at least one other category). ANOVA $F = 0.0486$ followed by LSD test ($p < 0.05$). Statistical analysis performed on log transformed data (not shown) as the original data was not normally distributed (Clarke *et al.*, 1993).

Results

Two protein bands of high apparent molecular mass (≥ 100 kDa) were identified in VCSF by immunoblotting with the various antibodies used to examine the brain fractions. These species had the approximate molecular mass of ≥ 116 and ≥ 125 kDa, and are likely to contain APP_{695} and APP_{KPI} (or derivatives), respectively. Only the band of highest molecular mass reacted strongly with all antibodies, including a KPI antibody (7H5), confirming that this species had the characteristics of APP_{KPI}.

The mean VCSF APP_{KPI} value determined with antibody 22C11 (Table 5) for patients receiving both lithium and antidepressants was significantly lower than that of patients receiving neither. This was not the case for APP_{695} although the difference in values between control and combination therapy was only slightly smaller in magnitude. The four treatment groups did not show any significant differences in age, sex, diagnostic group, or treatment with drugs of other categories. Results with the other antibodies confirmed the direction of changes seen with 22C11. However, the changes were most obvious with the other antibodies, including the β-amyloid protein antibody, 10D5.

Implications

These patients, whose illness was unresponsive to psychotropic drugs, showed evidence of differences in efflux of APP species from the brain that was dependent on the drugs that had been prescribed. The lowest value following treatment was with drugs that are likely either to interfere with PIP_2 recycling or inhibit neuronal activity by other, possibly similar, mechanisms. The most straightforward explanation of the present results is that these drugs inhibit α-secretase (Figure 1). This would reduce the secretion of non-amyloidogenic APP derivatives of high apparent molecular mass, probably from cortical pyramidal neurons which are subject to regulation by the appropriate receptors (Figure 3). Moreover, the reduction we have observed is in contrast to the finding that bradykinin, which activates PIP_2 breakdown, and phorbol esters, which mimic such hydrolysis, both stimulate secretion of APP-like immunoreactivity from PC12 cells (Table 1).

SUMMARY AND CONCLUSIONS

Figure 1 shows that a substantial loss of cortical cholinergic nerve endings, along with a much more circumscribed cortical degeneration of pyramidal neurons, almost certainly causes glutamatergic hypoactivity in living patients with AD. This would be exacerbated by the inhibitory action on these neurons of GABA interneurons and 5-HT, the latter effect mediated by the 5-HT_{1A} receptor. These transmitter abnormalities, with the exception of acetylcholine, probably also underlie DFT and Pick's disease (Table 2). In contrast, the cholinergic abnormality seems to be the major deficit in dementia of the Lewy body type. On the basis of current knowledge it is likely that a cholinomimetic will be useful in the treatment of all these disorders.

The use of volkensin as described here demonstrates that it is possible to selectively lesion subpopulations of cortical pyramidal neurons. This has allowed receptor changes to be ascribed to the loss of a specific type of cortical neuron, which has previously been impossible. The study has emphasized the importance of m_1 receptors for regulating pyramidal neuron activity (Table 3, Figure 3) underlining cognitive processes (Figure 2). Counts of these neurons in human neocortex correlate with apparent APP_{KPI} immunoreactivity which is particularly high in human compared with rat brain (Moir *et al.*, 1992). Table 4 shows that in the soluble fraction of the neocortex, the KPI insert appears to be predominantly in APP whereas in the high density membranes (presumably derived predominantly from the cell membrane of pyramidal neurons), it seems to be present in the APP homologue, APPH (Sprecher *et al.*, 1993; Wasco *et al.*, 1993). This observation may have important implications for the pathogenesis of AD as APPH does not contain an intact β-amyloid protein sequence. Thus it is important to study APPH as well as APP with respect to stimulation of the m_1 receptor.

It is well known that assessment of treatments designed to slow progression of pathology in AD will require study of many subjects over a long time period. Likewise, the prominent strategy relies on developing novel inhibitors for correcting suspected abnormal proteolysis of APP which is at present very poorly understood. This emphasizes the importance of discovering any role that currently understood receptors and available drugs may have in regulating metabolism of APP. The present data suggests that traditional pharmacological approaches being developed for the symptomatic treatment of AD (e.g. enhancing cholinergic transmission with agonists or acetylcholinesterase inhibitors (Davis *et al.*, 1992) are likely to affect selectively and positively the α-secretase processing pathway for APP (Figure 1). This pathway cannot lead to senile plaque formation and this treatment is likely to restore secretion (Francis *et al.*, 1993c) and maintain the extracellular supply of APP (or derivatives) apparently necessary for normal brain function.

Pharmacological treatment of AD is likely to be difficult both because of the presence of multiple transmitter changes and the difficulty of replacing lost transmitter function in a way that mimics normal neuronal release. With regard to the latter problem the introduction of agents which modify the actions of remaining transmitters may be a more effective approach than one based on the introduction of direct agonists. Most clinical studies to date have been directed towards the cholinergic deficit but acetylcholinesterase inhibitors that are ideal (i.e. long-lasting and non-toxic) have not yet emerged.

More studies are also needed on the neurobiology of APP, in particular of the extracellular function and its role in transmitter transduction mechanisms (Nishimoto *et al.*, 1993; see also Pearce and Potter, 1991; O'Neill *et al.*, 1991; McLaughlin *et al.*, 1991; Blier *et al.* 1992). However, drugs that affect transmission (Bowen, 1990; Francis *et al.*, 1993c) would now seem an important goal. These will be required for most patients to improve if not reverse functional cognitive disabilities already present, as well as for sufferers during the development of what are currently considered alternative non-transmitter related strategies. On the basis of the present discussion our working hypothesis is that drugs, such as acetylcholinesterase inhibitors, may also affect beneficially the metabolism of APP in the brain of patients with AD and influence the deposition of other proteins (tau and apolipoprotein E) implicated in sporadic AD. Further work may link receptor-mediated activity of pyramidal neurons to these proteins as well as to neurofibrillary tangle formation and neuronal loss (Figure 3).

ACKNOWLEDGEMENTS

We thank J. T. Alder, Dr N. A. Clarke, Dr C. Holmes, A. Misra and G. C. Stratmann for carrying out some of the assays and Drs

M. M. Esiri, D. M. A. Mann, R. Perry and Professors P. Lantos and N. Leigh for help in the collection and classification of some samples. We also thank Professor B. W. Agranoff for helpful advice and Drs D. Allsop and D. Schenk for antibodies.

Note added in proof

Tacrine is currently unique as it has passed the US Food and Drug administrations licensing procedure for use in treatment of mild to moderate Alzheimer's disease. It has also been approved by the authorities in France (Bowen, D.M., A start for Alzheimer's, *New Statesman & Society* 7 No 302, 27, 1994). However, the clinical response rates in those studies showing a modest benefit range between 3 and 50% (Bryne E., Arie, T., Tetrahydroaminoacridine and Alzheimer's disease, *Br. Med. J.* 868–869, 1994). Attributing this variability to a clinical factor such as a firm diagnosis of AD requires neuropathological confirmation. By contrast, we have argued (above) that two degenerative dementias, without apparent cholinergic dysfunction, may respond to tacrine. Levy and colleagues' recent work, as is well known, raised the suggestion that tacrine is mainly of benefit for another condition (Lewy body dementia). In some clinical trials cases of these dementias could have been inadvertently included and responded. It is unlikely that these rarer dementias have appreciably complicated trials with adequate numbers of patients. There is already evidence to support this as 3 out of 7 autopsy confirmed cases of AD 'responded' to tacrine (improved or stabilized cognitive ability or activities of daily living score) and a further case responded initially (G. K. Wilcock and M. I. Scott, personal communication). Li *et al.* have reiterated that impaired m_1 receptor responses may help to explain the limited therapeutic effect of cholinomimetics (Li, X., Song, L., Jope, R. S., Powers, R., Impaired cholinergic muscarinic receptor stimulated phosphoinositide hydrolysis in Alzheimer's disease, *Soc. Neurosci. Abs. 19*, 423, 1993). This group and Flynn *et al.* (above) apparently did not consider patients' immediate preterminal state. Allowance for this has now been made in our study of carbachol/GTP stimulation of phosphoinositide hydrolysis (assayed as described: Jope, R. S., Song, L., Powers, R., Agonist-induced, GTP-dependent phosphoinositide hydrolysis in postmortem human brain membranes, *J. Neurochem.* 62, 1–7, 1994). Under these conditions hydrolysis was dependent on calcium concentration and duration of terminal coma (I. P. Chessell, J. T. Alder and D. M. Bowen, unpublished observations). It is therefore important to consider these factors when comparing AD and control cases. Thus an impairment of m_1 responses may only occur in the event that the amount of calcium becomes rate-limiting. These considerations suggest that the variable and limited response to tacrine is related to errors in clinical trials (e.g. too few patients) and structural changes that co-exist (e.g. extent in degeneration of cholinergic and subpopulations of glutamatergic neurons). In conclusion, those deciding on the direction of drug development should persevere with the aim of improving activity of the remaining circuits of glutamatergic neurons (Figures 2 and 3) with cholinomimetrics, possibly in combination with a 5-HT_{1A} antagonist (Francis *et al.*, 1993b).

REFERENCES

Agranoff, B. W. (1989) Phosphoinositides in G. Siegel, B. Agranoff, R. W. Albers, and P. Molinoff (eds), *Basic Neurochemistry*, pp. 333–347. Raven Press, New York.

Berridge, M. J. (1993) Inositol trisphosphate and calcium signalling. *Nature*, **361**, 315–325.

Blier, P., Lista, A., and Montigny, C. D. (1992) Differential properties of pre- and postsynaptic 5-hydroxytryptamine$_{1A}$ receptors in the dorsal raphe and hippocampus: 11. Effect of pertussis and cholera toxins. *J. Pharmacol. Exp. Ther.*, **265**, 16–23.

Bowen, D. M. (1990) Treatment of Alzheimer's disease: Molecular pathology versus neurotransmitter-based therapy. *Br. J. Psychiatry*, **157**, 327–330.

Braak, H., and Braak, E. (1985) On areas of transition between entorhinal allocortex and temporal isocortex in the human brain. Normal morphology and lamina-specific pathology in Alzheimer's disease. *Act Neuropathol.*, **68**, 325–332.

Buckley, N. J., and Burnstock, G. (1986) Autoradiographic localisation of peripheral M1 muscarinic receptors using 3H pirenzepine. *Brain Res.*, **375**, 83–91.

Buxbaum, J. D., Oishi, M., Chen, H. I., Pinkas-Kramarski, P., Jaffe, E. A., Gandy, S. E., and Greengard, P. (1992) Cholinergic agonists and interleukin 1 regulate processing and secretion of the Alzheimer β/A4 amyloid protein precursor. *Proc. Natl Acad. Sci. USA*, **89**, 10075–10078.

Chessell, I. P., Francis, P. T., Pangalos, M. N., Pearson, R. C. A., and Bowen, D. M. (1993) Localisation of muscarinic (m_1) and other neurotransmitter receptors on corticofugal-projecting pyramidal neurones. *Brain Res.*, **632**, 86–94.

Chessell, I. P., Francis, P. T., Webster, M–T., Procter, A. W., Heath, P. R., Pearson, R. C. A., and Bowen, D. M. (1994) An aspect of Alzheimer neuropathology after suicide-transport damage. *J. Neural Transm.*, in press.

Clarke, N. A., Webster, M–T., Francis, P. T., Procter, A. W., Hodgkiss, A. D., and Bowen, D. M. (1993) β-Amyloid precursor protein-like immunoreactivity can be altered in humans by drugs affecting neurotransmitter function. *Neurodegeneration*, **2**, 243–248.

Court, J. A., and Perry, E. K. (1991) Dementia: The neurochemical basis of putative transmitter orientated therapy. *Pharmacol. Ther.*, **52**, 423–443.

Cowburn, R. F., O'Neil, C., Ravid, R., Alafuzoff, I., Winblad, B., and Fowler, C. J. (1992) Adenylyl cyclase activity in postmortem human brain: Evidence of altered G protein mediation in Alzheimer's disease. *J. Neurochem.*, **58**, 1409–1419.

Davis, K. L., Thal, L. J., Gamzu, E. R., Davis, C. S., Woolson, R. F., Gracon, S. I., Drachman, D. A., Schneider, L. S., Whitehouse, P. J., Hoover, T. M., Morris, J. C., Kawas, C. H., Knopman, D. S., Earl, N. L., Kumar, V., and Doody, R. S. (1992) A double-blind, placebo-controlled multicenter study of tacrine for Alzheimer's disease. *N. Engl. J. Med.*, **327**, 1253–1259.

DeKosky, S. T., and Scheff, S. W. (1990) Synapse loss in frontal cortex biopsies in Alzheimer's disease: correlation with cognitive severity. *Ann. Neurol.*, **27**, 457–464.

Francis, P. T., Pangalos, M. N., and Bowen, D. M. (1992a) Animal and drug modelling for Alzheimer synaptic pathology. *Prog. Neurobiol.*, **39**, 517–545.

Francis, P. T., Pangalos, M. N., Pearson, R. C. A., Middlemiss, D. N., Stratmann, G. C., and Bowen, D. M. (1992b) 5-HT_{1A} but not 5-HT_2 receptors are enriched on neocortical pyramidal neurones destroyed by intrastriatal volkensin. *J. Pharmacol. Exp. Ther.*, **261**, 1273–1281.

Francis, P. T., Cross, A. J., and Bowen, D. M. (1994) Neurotransmitters and neuropeptides, in R. D. Terry, R. Katzman, and K. Bick (eds), *Alzheimer Disease*, pp 247–261, Raven Press, New York.

Francis, P. T., Holmes, C., Webster, M–T., Stratmann, G. C., Procter, A. W., and Bowen, D. M. (1993a) Preliminary neurochemical findings in non-Alzheimer dementia due to lobar atrophy. *Dementia*, **4**, 172–177.

Francis, P. T., Sims, N. R., Procter, A. W., and Bowen, D. M. (1993b) Cortical pyramidal neurone loss may cause glutamatergic hypoactivity and cognitive impairment in Alzheimer's disease: investigative and therapeutic perspectives. *J. Neurochem.*, **60**, 1589–1604.

Francis, P. T., Webster, M–T., Procter, A. W., Clark, N. A., Bowen, D. M., Doshi, R., Mann, D. M. A., and Neary, D. (1993c) Soluble β-amyloid precursor protein and pyramidal neurone loss. *Lancet*, **341**, 431.

Fukushima, D., Konishi, M., Maruyama, K., Miyamoto, T., Ishiura, S., and Suzuki, K. (1993) Activation of the α secretory pathway leads to a decrease in the intracellular amyloidogenic fragments generated from the amyloid protein precursor. *Biochem. Biophys. Res. Commun.*, **194**, 202–207.

Haass, C., Hung, A. Y., and Selkoe, D. J. (1991) Processing of β-amyloid precursor protein in microglia and astrocytes favors an internal localization over constitutive secretion. *J. Neurosci.*, **11**, 3783–3793.

Hansen, L., Salmon, D., Galasko, D., Masliah, E., Katzman, R., DeTeresa, R., Thal, L., Pay, M. M., Hofstetter, R., Klauber, M., Rice, V., Butters, N., and Alford, M. (1990) The Lewy body variant of Alzheimer's disease: A clinical and pathologic entity. *Neurology*, **40**, 1–8.

Hulme, E. C., Birdsall, N. J. M., and Buckley, N. J. (1990) Muscarinic receptor subtypes. *Annu. Rev. Pharmacol. Toxicol.*, **30**, 633–673.

Kesslak, J. P., Nalcioglu, O., and Cotman, C. W. (1991) Quantification of magnetic resonance scans for hippocampal and parahippocampal atrophy in Alzheimer's disease. *Neurology*, **41**, 51–54.

Kowall, N. W., and Beal, M. F. (1991) Glutamate-, glutaminase-, and taurine-immunoreactive neurones develop neurofibrillary tangles in Alzheimer's disease. *Ann. Neurol.*, **29**, 162–167.

Lewis, D. A., Campbell, M. J., Terry, R. D., and Morrison, J. H. (1987) Laminar and regional distributions of neurofibrillary tangles and neuritic plaques in Alzheimer's disease: a quantitative study of visual and auditory cortices. *J. Neurosci.*, **7**, 1799–1809.

Madhok, T. C. (1993) Nerve growth factor enhances [^{3}H]nicotine binding to a nicotinic cholinergic receptor on PC 12 cells. *Endocrinology*, **130**, 825–830.

Mann, D. M. A., South, P. W., Snowden, J. S., and Neary, D. (1993) Dementia of frontal lobe type: neuropathology and immunohistochemistry. *J. Neurol. Neurosurg. Psychiatry*, **56**, 605–614.

McCormick, D. A., and Williamson, A. (1989) Convergence and divergence of neurotransmitter action in human cerebral cortex. *Proc. Natl Acad. Sci. USA*, **86**, 8098–8102.

McLaughlin, M., Ross, B.M., Milligan, G., McCulloch, J., and Knowler, J. T. (1991) Robustness of G proteins in Alzheimer's disease: An immunoblot study. *J. Neurochem.*, **57**, 9–14.

Moir, R. D., Martin, R. N., Bush, A. I., Small, D. H., Milward, E. A., Rumble, B. A., Multhaup, G., Beyreuther, K., and Master, C. L. (1992) Human brain βA4 amyloid protein precursor of Alzheimer's disease: Purification and partial characterization. *J. Neurochem.*, **59**, 1490–1498.

Neary, D., Snowden, J. S., Mann, D. M., Bowen, D. M., Sims, N. R., Northen, B., Yates, P. O., and Davison, A. N. (1986) Alzheimer's disease: a correlative study. *J. Neurol. Neurosurg. Psychiatry*, **49**, 229–237.

Neary, D., Snowden, J. S., and Mann, D. M. A. (1993) The clinical pathological correlates of lobar atrophy. *Dementia*, **4**, 154–159.

Nishimoto, I., Okamoto, T., Matsuura, Y., Takahashi, S., Okamoto, T. O., Murayama, Y., and Ogata, E. (1993) Alzheimer amyloid protein precursor complexes with brain GTP-binding protein G_0. *Nature*, **362**, 75–79.

Nitsch, R. M., Slack, B. E., Wurtman, R. J., and Growdon, J. H. (1992) Release of Alzheimer amyloid precursor stimulated by activation of muscarinic acetylcholine receptors. *Science*, **258**, 304–307.

Nitsch, R. M., Farber, S. A., Growdon, J. H., and Wurtman, R. J. (1993) Release of amyloid β-protein precursor derivatives by electrical depolarization of rat hippocampal slices. *Proc. Natl Acad. Sci. USA*, **90**, 5191–5193.

O'Neill, C., Cowburn, R. F., Wiehager, B., Alafuzoff, I., Winblad, B., and Fowler, C. J. (1991) Preservation of 5-hydroxytryptamine$_{1A}$ receptor–G protein interactions in the cerebral cortex of patients with Alzheimer's disease. *Neurosci. Lett.*, **133**, 15–19.

Pangalos, M. N., Francis, P. T., Middlemiss, D. N., Pearson, R. C. A., and Bowen, D. M. (1991) Selective destruction of a sub-population of cortical neurones by suicide transport of volkensin, a lectin from Adenia volkensii. *J. Neurosci. Methods*, **40**, 17–29.

Pangalos, M. N., Francis, P. T., Foster, A. C., Pearson, R. C. A., Middlemiss, D. N., and Bowen, D. M. (1992) NMDA receptors assessed by autoradiography with [^{3}H] L-689,560 are present but not enriched on corticofugal-projecting pyramidal neurones. *Brain Res.*, **596**, 223–230.

Pearce, B. D., and Potter, L. T. (1991) Coupling of m1 muscarinic receptors to G protein in Alzheimer disease. *Alzheimer Dis. Assoc. Disord.*, **5**, 163–172.

Pearson, R. C. A., Esiri, M. M., Hiorns, R. W., Wilcock, G. K., and Powell, T. P.S. (1985) Anatomical correlates of the distribution of the pathological changes in the neocortex in Alzheimer's disease. *Proc. Natl Acad. Sci. USA*, **82**, 4531–4534.

Perry, E. K., Kerwin, J. M., Perry, R. H., Irving, D., Blessed, G., and Fairbairn, A. F. (1990) Cerebral cholinergic activity is related to the incidence of visual hallucinations in senile dementia of Lewy body type. *Dementia*, **1**, 2–4.

Poulter, L., Barratt, D., Scott, C. W., and Caputo, C. B. (1993) Locations of immunoreactivities of phosphorylation sites on bovine and porcine tau proteins and a PHF-Tau fragment. *J. Biol. Chem.*, **268**, 9636–9644.

Procter, A. W., Doshi, R., Bowen, D. M., and Murphy, E. (1990) Rapid autopsy brains for biochemical research: experiences in establishing a programme. *Int. J. Geriatr. Psychiatry*, **5**, 287–294.

Saunders, A. M., Stritmatter, W. J., Schmechel, D., St. George-Heslop, P. H., Pericak-Vance, M. A., Joo, S. H., Rosi, B. L., Gusella, J. F., Crapper-MacLachlan, D. R., Alberts, M. J., Hulette, C., Crain, B., Goldgaber, D., and Roses, A. D. (1993) Association of apolipoprotein E allele E4 with late-onset familial and sporadic Alzheimer's disease. *Neurology*, **43**, 1467–1472.

Schoepp, D. D., and True, R. A. (1992) 1*S*,3*R*-ACPD-sensitive (metabotropic) [^{3}H]glutamate receptor binding in membranes. *Neurosci. Lett.*, **145**, 100–104.

Shigematsu, K., McGeer, P. L., and McGeer, E. G. (1992) Localization of amyloid precursor protein in selective postsynaptic densities of rat cortical neurons. *Brain Res.*, **592**, 353–357.

Sinha, S., and Lieberburg, I. (1992) Normal metabolism of the amyloid precursor protein (APP). *Neurodegeneration*, **1**, 169–175.

Sparks, L. D., Hunsaker, J. C., Slevin, J. T., DeKosky, S. T., Kryscio, R. J., and Markesbery, W. R. (1992) Monoaminergic and cholinergic synaptic markers in the nucleus basalis of Meynert (nbM): Normal age-related changes and the effect of heart disease and Alzheimer's disease. *Ann. Neurol.*, **31**, 611–620.

Sprecher, C. A., Grant, F. J., Grimm, G., O'Hara, P. J., Norris, F., Norris, K., and Foster, D. C. (1993) Molecular cloning of the cDNA for a human amyloid precursor protein homolog: Evidence for a multigene family. *Biochemistry*, **32**, 4481–4486.

Steele, J. E., Cross, A. J., and Bowen, D. M. (1992) *N*-methyl-D-aspartate receptor-associated ionophores determined in Alzheimer's disease by [^{3}H]MK-801 and *N*-[1-(2-thienyl)cyclohexyl]-3,4-[^{3}H]piperidine binding. *Neurodegeneration*, **1**, 225–230.

Stubbs, E. B., and Agranoff, B. W. (1993) Lithium enhances muscarinic receptor-stimulated CDP-diacylglycerol formation in inositol-depleted SK-N-SH neuroblastoma cells. *J. Neurochem.*, **60**, 1292–1299.

Terry, R. D., Masliah, E., Salmon, D. P., Butters, N., DeTeresa, R., Hill, R., Hansen, L. A., and Katzman, R. (1991) Physical basis of cognitive alterations in Alzheimer's disease: synapse loss is the major correlate of cognitive impairment. *Ann. Neurol.*, **30**, 572–580.

Wasco, W., Gurubhagavatula, S., Paradis, M. D., Romario, D. M., Sisodia, S. S., Hyman, B. T., Neve, R. L., and Tanzi, R. E. (1993) Isolation and characterization of the human APLP2 gene encoding a homologue of the Alzheimer's associated amyloid β protein precursor. *Nature Genet.*, **5**, 95–100.

Webster, M–T., Francis, P. T., Procter, A. W., Stratmann, G. C., Doshi, R., Mann, D. M. A., and Bowen, D. M. (1994) Postmortem brains reveal similar but not identical APP-like immunoreactivity in Alzheimer compared with other dementias. *Brain Res.*, **644**, 347–351.

Webster, M–T., Vekrellis, K., Francis, P. T., Pearce, B. R., and Bowen, D. M. (1993) Factors affecting the β-amyloid precursor in PC12 cells. *Biochem. Soc. Trans.*, **21**, 239S.

Wiley, R. G. (1992) Neural lesioning with ribosome-inactivating proteins: suicide transport and immunolesioning. *Trends. Neurosci.*, **15**, 285–290.

Zilles, K., Gross, G., Schleicher, A., Schildgen, S., Bauer, A., Bahro, M., Schwendemann, G., Zech, K., and Kolassa, N. (1991) Regional and laminar distributions of α_1-adrenoceptors and their subtypes in human and rat hippocampus. *Neuroscience*, **40**, 307–320.

7

β-Amyloid, Cytokines and Other Potential Strategies for Modifying the Pathophysiology of Alzheimer's Disease

C. A. Wilmot, S. R. Sahasrabudhe, G. E. Ringheim, L. L. Martin, and R. C. Effland

Neuroscience Strategic Business Unit, Hoechst-Roussel Pharmaceuticals, Inc., Somerville, NJ, USA

A current challenge for neuroscience research and the pharmaceutical industry is the discovery and development of therapeutics for the treatment of Alzheimer's disease (AD), a disabling neurodegenerative disorder with increasing incidence in the aging population. Since the observation of significant losses of cholinergic neurons in postmortem brains of AD patients (Whitehouse *et al.*, 1981), drug discovery efforts have focused on restoring these deficits through cholinergic mechanisms of action, such as inhibition of acetylcholinesterase, muscarinic receptor agonists or the facilitation of acetylcholine release (Smith and Swash, 1978; Collerton, 1986; Fibiger, 1991). The aminoacridine cholinesterase inhibitor Cognex® (tacrine) representative of this first generation of therapeutics, have provided symptomatic benefits (Davis *et al.*, 1992; Farlow *et al.*,

Alzheimer's Disease: Clinical and Treatment Perspectives. Edited by N. R. Cutler, C. G. Gottfries and K. Siegfried.

1992). However, the modest degree of improvement and the potential for side-effects will probably limit their use. Alternative pharmacological approaches, e.g. restoration of other neurotransmitter deficits, nootropics, CNS stimulants and vasodilators, are also being explored but have not been highly successful (Miller *et al.*, 1992b). Unfortunately, while providing some benefit for the cognitive and behavioral deficits, symptomatic treatments do not affect the underlying pathophysiology.

As our understanding of the pathophysiology of AD advances, a second generation of therapeutics with mechanisms of action targeted to the neurodegenerative processes could provide palliative treatments to retard disease progression or curative effects to halt the process itself. The scope of this chapter is to review several mechanistic strategies for new therapeutics targeted at the pathophysiology of AD including interventions with amyloid plaque formation, immune-mediated mechanisms and free radical induced damage contributing to the brain pathology.

ALZHEIMER'S DISEASE CELLULAR PATHOLOGY

Our knowledge of AD pathophysiology is presently limited to the postmortem diagnostic histology characterized by senile amyloid plaques, neurofibrillary tangles (NFT) and neuronal loss (Dickson *et al.*, 1988). Senile plaques are complex extracellular depositions, of which the major proteinaceous component is β-amyloid (βA4), a 39–42 amino acid peptide (Glenner and Wong, 1984). Other proteins associated with or identified within plaques include α_1-antichymotrypsin, ubiquitin, apolipoprotein E (ApoE), acetylcholinesterase, and tyrosine hydroxylase. Dystrophic neurites are also found within the plaques. NFT are insoluble fibrils, primarily of paired helical filaments (PHF) formed from microtubule-associated tau proteins, which accumulate intracellularly in degenerating neurons and in dystrophic neurites surrounding the senile plaques (Goedert, 1993). Whether or not the formation of the neuritic amyloid plaques and neurofibrillary tangles are part of the disease etiology or are the result of a neurodegenerative process is not clear (Selkoe, 1991).

Microglia or brain macrophages are also prominent in the brain lesions (Cras *et al.*, 1990, 1991; Perlmutter *et al.*, 1990). Mature senile plaques are surrounded by microglia which extend their processes into the core plaque areas (Haga *et al.*, 1989; McGeer *et al.*, 1988). These microglia appear to be activated, displaying an ameboid phagocytic morphology in contrast to the ramified non-activated form characterized by long, extended processes. The observation that plaque-associated microglia also display surface antigens (HLA-DR) is an indicator of the immunological activation of these cells (McGeer *et al.*, 1987, 1989; Perlmutter *et al.*, 1992). The stimulating factors for this activation are unknown but may be specific proteins found in plaque cores. For example, laminin, a component of plaques, can induce the transformation of ramified microglia to a rounded phagocytic form in cell culture (Charmak and Mallat, 1991). In addition, βA4 has been reported to stimulate proliferation of microglia in culture (Araujo and Cotman, 1992). The prominence of microglia at the lesion site may therefore be a result of local infiltration and proliferation, though chemotactic recruitment of additional macrophages into the region cannot be ruled out. Microglia-derived cytotoxic products and other secretory factors may contribute to the progression of the pathology (Nakajima and Kohsaka, 1993; Perry *et al.*, 1993).

The loss of cholinergic neurons in the basal forebrain nucleus of Meynert has been implicated in the cognitive decline due to the extensive cholinergic projections of these neurons to the hippocampus and cerebral cortex and the well established experimental evidence for a significant role of acetylcholine and these brain areas in learning and memory (Bartus *et al.*, 1982; Fibiger, 1991; Holttum and Gershon, 1992). However, there are also significant losses of neurons in the hippocampus, cortico-cortical association pathways (possibly glutamatergic), locus coeruleus noradrenergic neurons and brain stem serotonergic raphe neurons (Gottfries, 1985; Struble *et al.*, 1987; Bowen, 1988; Palmer and Gershon, 1990; Chan-Palay, 1990). Thus, multiple neurotransmitter deficits are postulated to contribute not only to the cognitive deficits but also the behavioral disturbances in AD patients. With the high prevalence of cortical and hippocampal pathology, it has been proposed that the primary lesion may be cortical, with secondary effects on subcortical neurons

(Armstrong, 1993; DeLacoste and White, 1993). Although the temporal progression of the neuronal losses and the relationship to the plaque and tangle histopathology are not known, a central role for βA4 has been widely speculated (Katzman and Saitoh, 1991; Yankner and Mesulam, 1991; Hardy and Higgins, 1992).

βA4 AND THE MOLECULAR PATHOLOGY

The hypothesis that accelerated βA4 deposition is an early and critical event in the development of AD continues to gain support from studies in cultured cells, animals and humans (Selkoe, 1993). Support for a causal relationship for βA4 and AD is derived from several sources: (1) a positive correlation of plaque density and dementia (Hyman *et al.*, 1993); (2) identification of mutations in the amyloid precursor protein (APP) in familial AD (Ashall and Goate, 1994); (3) the association of Down's syndrome neuropathology and symptoms with the overexpression of the APP gene on chromosome 21 (Masters *et al.*, 1985a, 1985b); and (4) experimental evidence for βA4 neurotoxicity and potentiation of excitatory amino acid toxicity (Snow and Malouf, 1993). Although the total number of senile plaques and the total amyloid load are higher in AD patients compared to age-matched individuals, neither of these measures necessarily correlates with the duration of illness or severity of dementia (Arendt *et al.*, 1984; Mann *et al.*, 1985). Hyman *et al.* (1993) have therefore proposed that there may be a dynamic equilibrium between the rates of formation and destruction of amyloid that is disturbed in AD. The presence of NFT may also be a critical factor for the expression of AD, since amyloid plaques in the absence of NFT were not correlated with dementia in some studies (Braak and Braak, 1991).

The strongest evidence for involvement of APP in AD comes from studies of early onset familial AD. The familial mutations at codons 670 and 671, 692, 713, and 717 of APP-770 have been found to co-segregate with AD (Goate *et al.*, 1991; Murrell *et al.*, 1991; Chartier-Harlin *et al.*, 1991; Mullan *et al.*, 1992; Jones *et al.*, 1992). Only one of the mutations at codons 670 and 671 has been shown to increase secreted βA4 (Citron *et al.*, 1992; Cai *et al.*, 1992). Although only a small percentage (~5%) of the total AD population is accounted for by familial AD, these results suggest that mutations in the APP gene may cause the complete AD pathology. It is therefore possible that dysfunction in APP metabolism plays an important role in the disease.

The possibility of altering the disease process by interfering with the formation of βA4 from its precursor APP has led to considerable experimental investigation. Analysis of the cDNA clone isolated using oligonucleotides corresponding to the deduced peptide sequence revealed that βA4 was an internal proteolytic fragment of a larger protein encoded by a gene on chromosome 21 in band q21 (Kang *et al.*, 1987; Tanzi *et al.*, 1987; Goldgaber *et al.*, 1987; Robakis *et al.*, 1987). The APP gene is encoded by at least 18 exons and spans more than 170 kilo-bases (Yoshikai *et al.*, 1990). Several different alternatively spliced forms of APP, namely APP-695, APP-714, APP-751, APP-770, APP-563, and APP-365, have been reported (Ashall and Goate, 1994). APP-695, 751, and 770 are integral membrane glycoproteins containing a large extracytoplasmic domain, a transmembrane domain and a small cytoplasmic sequence. The first 28 amino acid residues of βA4 are extracellular and the last 14 residues are within the transmembrane domain. The βA4 sequence arises from parts of exons 16 and 17 (using APP-770 numbering) and therefore cannot be generated by alternate splicing. The isoforms APP-751 and APP-770 contain a 56 amino acid insert homologous to the Kunitz family of protease inhibitors (KPI) (Kitaguchi *et al.*, 1988; Tanzi *et al.*, 1988). APP-770 also contains a 19 amino acid insert homologous to the OX-2 antigen, a protein present in neurons and thymocytes (Kitaguchi *et al.*, 1988). A novel alternatively spliced form of APP which excludes exon 15 has been reported in T-lymphocytes, macrophages and microglia (Konig *et al.*, 1992).

Although the physiological roles of APP in the brain are unclear, it has been implicated in the growth, repair, intracellular trafficking of proteins and cell adhesion. APP is a highly conserved molecule present in almost all tissues and cell lines. APP synthesis is up-regulated in response to ischemia, trauma, toxic agents and interruption of nerve impulse flow (Abe *et al.*, 1991; Kawarabayashi *et al.*, 1991; Wallace *et al.*, 1991; Shigematsu and McGeer, 1992; Stephenson *et al.*, 1992; Wakita *et al.*, 1992; Gentleman *et al.*, 1993; Wallace *et al.*, 1993). Head injury has been identified as a risk factor for AD, and increased production of APP and generation of βA4 may be part of its biochemical basis (Henderson, 1988; Graves *et al.*, 1990).

METABOLISM OF APP

Newly synthesized APP undergoes several post-translational modifications including N- and O-linked glycosylation, tyrosine sulfation, phosphorylation and secretion of the extracellular domain (Weidemann *et al.*, 1989; Oltersdorf *et al.*, 1990; Refolo *et al.*, 1989) The KPI-containing isoforms of APP may also occur as the core of chondroitin sulfate proteoglycan (Shioi *et al.*, 1992). APP-secretase (α-secretase) is a hypothetical enzyme that cleaves the full length APP between amino acids Lys-16 and Leu-17 of the βA4 sequence (Esch *et al.*, 1990; Sisodia *et al.*, 1990; Anderson *et al.*, 1991). This non-amyloidogenic cleavage prevents the production of βA4 and results in the secretion of the large extracellular domain of APP. Alteration in secretase activity may therefore influence the amount of amyloid formed. Mutagenesis of the region surrounding the secretase site does not result in any significant alteration in secretase activity (Maruyama *et al.*, 1991; Sisodia, 1992). Secretase cleavage occurs approximately 12 amino acids amino-terminal to the beginning of the trans-membrane domain in a variety of sequence contexts (Sahasrabudhe *et al.*, 1992). Phorbol esters, cholinergic agonists, muscarinic receptors and nerve growth factor regulate the activity of secretase in cell cultures (Caporaso *et al.*, 1992; Buxbaum *et al.*, 1992; Nitsch *et al.*, 1992; Refolo *et al.*, 1989). In cultured cells, APP present on the plasma membrane are subjected to secretase cleavage (Sisodia, 1992; Haass *et al.*, 1992a; Sahasrabudhe *et al.*, 1992). However, secretase-cleaved APP has also been recovered in the internal membrane vesicles of PC-12 cells prior to release into the medium, suggesting that the cleavage may take place in the trans-Golgi compartment before APP reaches the plasma membrane (Sambamurti *et al.*, 1992). Thus, depending on the cell type, secretase cleavage may take place in both trans-Golgi vesicles and the plasma membrane to varying extents.

Since βA4 was detected in senile plaques, it was assumed that this peptide was the result of abnormal cleavage of APP. It has now been shown that βA4 is continuously generated *in vivo* as well as in the conditioned medium of cells expressing APP (Haass *et al.*, 1992b; Seubert *et al.*, 1992; Shoji *et al.*, 1992). The normally produced βA4 peptides (in conditioned medium of cells expressing APP) have heterogeneous amino termini at Ile-6, Val-3, Asp-1, Phe-4 or Glu-11 (Haass *et al.*, 1992b; Seubert *et al.*, 1992; Busciglio *et al.*, 1993). The human cerebrospinal fluid (CSF) contains βA4 peptides ending at residue numbers 27, 28, 30, 34, 35, 40, 43 (Vigo-Pilfrey, 1993), whereas a majority of soluble peptides obtained from cells in culture end at residue 40 (Haass *et al.*, 1992b; Seubert *et al.*, 1992). βA4 peptides are secreted by unidentified cellular mechanisms before they can accumulate intracellularly.

It is not clear if the normally produced βA4 peptides found in the conditioned medium of cells expressing APP or in the plasma and CSF are also the ones present in senile plaques. The plaque amyloid as well as the vascular amyloid found in AD tissue do not show the type of heterogeneity found in normally secreted βA4 peptides (Miller *et al.*, 1992a; Masters *et al.*, 1985a, b). Plaque amyloid also contains peptides 75–85 residues long which comprise the entire sequence of βA4 and additional amino acids from the carboxy-terminus of APP (Miller *et al.*, 1993). It is, however, possible that at least some of the plaque peptides result from limited proteolysis of the normally secreted peptides. Alternatively, the plaque peptides may be formed after the internalization of βA4 peptide within lysosomes (Knauer *et al.*, 1992) and subsequently released after neuronal death.

Amyloid deposits may arise not only from an abnormal increase in the concentration of βA4 but also from the aggregation of the peptide in brain. Thus, therapeutic approaches solely aimed at blocking or decreasing the production of βA4 may have limitations. Since βA4 peptides are normally produced *in vivo*, they may have an unidentified important physiological role. It is not understood why the βA4 peptides formed in normal individuals do not aggregate. The reduced tendency of rodent amyloid to aggregate may be due to three amino acid substitutions, i.e. Arg-5, Tyr-10, and His-13, with respect to the human peptide sequence (Dyrks *et al.*, 1993) and reduced zinc-binding affinity (Bush *et al.*, 1994). Although the rate of aggregation of βA4 is slow in the absence of nucleating reagents, the presence of Ile-41 and Ala-42 increase the rate of aggregation by several fold (Jarrett *et al.*, 1993). Jarrett and Lansbury (1993) suggest that nucleation-dependent polymerization, the proposed mechanism of βA4 aggregation, can be prevented by reducing the βA4 concentration or by interfering with nucleus formation. Local pH, ionic strength zinc-binding and metal-catalyzed oxidation reactions may also play important roles in the aggregation process (Burdick *et al.*, 1992; Dyrks *et al.*, 1992; Bush *et al.*, 1994). Since free radical scavengers, ascorbic acid and trolox, have been shown to prevent βA4 aggregation, antioxidants and free radical scavengers may have therapeutic potential to retard the progression of the pathology (Dyrks *et al.*, 1992, 1993).

IN VIVO AND *IN VITRO* TOXICITY OF βA4

The neurotoxicity of βA4 as a contributing factor in AD has been widely debated. The neurotoxic activity seems to be specific to aggregated βA4 (Pike *et al.*, 1991, 1993). The mechanism by which the aggregated form exerts toxicity remains unclear, and both apoptosis and a destabilization of calcium homeostasis have been proposed (Loo *et al.*, 1993; Mattson *et al.*, 1992). There may be significant lot-to-lot variations of βA4 with respect to neurotoxicity to embryonic rat cells *in vitro* (May *et al.*, 1992; Fortes and Sahasrabudhe, unpublished results). Busciglio and Yankner (1992) showed that neurotoxic lots of monomeric βA4 exhibit a significant α-helix conformation by circular dichroism spectroscopy. Soluble βA4, on the other hand, may have beneficial biological functions, such as promotion of neurite extension or tachykinin receptor activation (Pike *et al.*, 1991; Kimura and Schubert, 1993).

Conflicting results have emerged from studies on the toxicity of βA4 *in vivo*. The initial *in vivo* studies with hippocampal or cortical infusion of synthetic βA4 or SDS-extracted amyloid cores derived from AD brains suggested a neurotoxic effect in rats (Kowall *et al.*, 1991; Frautschy *et al.*, 1991, 1992). Subsequent experiments, however, conflicted with these earlier results (Clemens and Stephenson, 1992; Emre *et al.*, 1992; Games *et al.*,

1992; Kowall *et al.*, 1992; Podlisny *et al.*, 1992; Rush *et al.*, 1992; Stein-Behrens *et al.*, 1992; Waite *et al.*, 1992). The discrepancies in these studies may in part be due to the aggregation status of the peptide and the concentration used. It is also extremely difficult to effectively deliver sufficient quantities of βA4 peptide *in vivo* because of its aggregation properties. Furthermore, *in vivo* toxicity of βA4 may depend on the presence of other factors, such as pathological chaperone molecules.

It is clear from the *in vitro* as well as some *in vivo* studies that the aggregated form of βA4 is the toxic component. It is also clear that in normal individuals βA4 does not aggregate despite being present in ng/ml concentrations. Physiological chaperone molecules have been postulated to prevent βA4 fibril formation based on evidence from studies on human CSF (Wisniewski *et al.*, 1993a). On the other hand, some molecules specific to AD pathology may promote the aggregation of βA4. ApoE, a plasma lipoprotein, was recently shown to be localized in senile plaques, congophilic angiopathy, and NFT of AD brains (Rebeck *et al.*, 1993; Strittmatter *et al.*, 1993a; Wisniewski *et al.*, 1993b). Individuals that inherit 2 alleles of ApoE4 are more likely (8 times) to have AD compared to normal individuals (Corder *et al.*, 1993). Autopsied brains of homozygous ApoE4 AD patients have greater congo red angiopathy and senile plaque staining compared to ApoE3 homozygotes (Strittmatter *et al.*, 1993a). Although both ApoE3 and ApoE4 isoforms form non-covalent SDS-resistant complexes with βA4, binding of βA4 to ApoE4 occurs within minutes rather than hours as for ApoE3 (Strittmatter *et al.*, 1993b). The presence of ApoE in NFT suggests that an ApoE–βA4 complex may be internalized by neurons (Strittmatter *et al.*, 1993a and b). Although the relevance of this binding to the pathophysiology remains to be established, modulation of these interactions may represent another target for therapeutic intervention.

βA4 BASED THERAPEUTIC APPROACHES

Many therapeutic approaches geared towards preventing the formation, aggregation or toxicity of βA4 have been proposed. βA4 formation can be halted or decreased by designing inhibitors of enzymes(s) that result in the formation of amino or carboxy terminus of βA4. Activations of α-secretase or kinases that result in increased cleavage of APP could prove to be effective amyloid inhibitors. Since aggregation of βA4 seems to be important for *in vivo* as well as *in vitro* toxicity, it may be useful to design molecules that prevent the initiating events in the aggregation process. The discovery of a compound that inhibits βA4 aggregation can be facilitated by the identification of key amino acid residues involved in the nucleating events that lead to the formation of an aggregate. Molecules that mimic the aforementioned peptides could serve as good leads for drug candidates.

IMMUNE-RELATED PATHOPHYSIOLOGY

Of clinical importance in AD is the elevation of brain immunological activity. For example, the cytokines IL-1 (Griffen *et al.*, 1989) and IL-6 (Strauss *et al.*, 1992) are elevated in the brain of Alzheimer's patients indicating that there is an active inflammatory response. In addition, immunoreactivity for the acute phase proteins α_1-antichymotrypsin (Abraham *et al.*, 1988; Rozemuller *et al.*, 1989) and α_2-macroglobulin (Strauss *et al.*, 1992) is associated with some areas of the pathology. Generally, production of acute phase proteins is associated with immune response activation, and in particular, a response to IL-1 and IL-6.

In addition to immunopathological processes, the presence of inflammatory cytokines and acute phase proteins also has implications regarding the expression and processing of APP. In PC-12 cells, both IL-1β (Buxbaum *et al.*, 1992) and IL-6 (Alstiel and Sperber, 1991) upregulate the amount of secreted APP fragments. Whether this is a result of total protein production, secretase activity, or both is not clear. IL-1β elevates APP gene transcription in cultured cells (Goldgaber *et al.*, 1989; Donnelly *et al.*, 1990). It has also been shown to stimulate the production of α_2-macroglobulin which inhibits the secretion of βA4 (Ganter *et al.*, 1991). Thus, cytokines may contribute to AD pathology by regulating APP gene expression and/or proteolytic processing, and may be new avenues for the control of βA4 formation.

Complement proteins are also present in AD brains (Eikelenboom *et al.*, 1982; McGeer *et al.*, 1989), implicating direct involvement of the immune system with the observed cellular pathology. Complement activity in the brain would appear at first glance to be restricted since serum proteins have difficulty crossing the blood–brain barrier. However, cells of astrocytic and neuronal origins (Walker and McGeer, 1993) as well as microglial origins (Haga *et al.*, 1993) can produce complement proteins *in vitro*. In AD brains, the relative abundance of mRNA for complement proteins C3 and C4 is increased three-fold relative to age-matched controls (Walker and McGeer, 1992). Thus, many of the components involved in the complement cascade may be produced locally in the brain. Regardless of the origin of the complement proteins, there is evidence that the C5b-9 membrane attack complex (MAC), the final stage in the complement-mediated cell lysis event, exists in association with dystrophic neurites, neuropil threads, and tangled neurons (McGeer *et al.*, 1989). A membrane inhibitor of complement-mediated reactive lysis (CD59 or MIRL) is also detected in AD brains in a pattern similar to the MAC complex, suggesting a compensatory up-regulation of a protective mechanism in response to complement-mediated neuronal injury (McGeer *et al.*, 1991). A role for complement in the progression of AD pathology is suggested by the observation that immunoreactivity for the MAC complex is present only in compacted plaques, but not diffuse plaques of the cerebellum (Lue and Rogers, 1992). In contrast to activation of the classical pathway for complement cascade by immunoglobulin, βA4 has been shown to bind and activate complement both *in vitro* and *in situ* with AD brain sections (Rogers *et al.*, 1992b). The association of these proteins with the pathology has led to the hypothesis that AD may be amenable to antiinflammatory therapeutic regimens (McGeer and Rogers, 1992).

CYTOKINE/IMMUNE-SYSTEM BASED THERAPEUTIC APPROACHES

A retrospective analysis of the incidence of AD in patients with rheumatoid arthritis and the converse provided support for the hypothesis that antiinflammatory agents may have a therapeutic effect (McGeer and Rogers, 1992). The estimated prevalence of

AD in rheumatoid arthritis clinics or in hospitals was approximately 0.4%, whereas the incidence in the general population of 64 years or older was estimated to be 2.4–10.3%. Conversely, in postmortem diagnosed AD patients, only two (of 290) individuals had a history of rheumatoid arthritis (0.7%). The implication from this analysis was that the two pathological conditions may be mutually exclusive, possibly due to the chronic use of antiinflammatory drugs by those affected with arthritis. A similar interpretation was made from the low incidence of AD in a population of isolated Japanese lepers treated with the antibacterial and antiinflammatory agent dapsone (McGeer *et al.*, 1992).

If cytokines and immune activation are causal or contributory factors to AD pathology, then compounds that regulate gene transcription of antiinflammatory or proinflammatory proteins may be of therapeutic value. In the case of proteins with antiinflammatory effects, upregulating gene expression may be desired. Conversely, in the case of proinflammatory proteins such as IL-1 and TNF-α, down-regulation of gene expression may be useful. Steroid compounds are commonly used for the treatment of inflammatory conditions and part of their usefulness may well be their strong inhibitory effects on proinflammatory cytokine gene transcription.

Following transcription, some proinflammatory proteins remain inactive until they are proteolytically processed. Inhibiting conversion of these proteins to active molecules represents an attractive point for drug intervention. IL-1β, for example, is first translated to an inactive 31 kDa precursor protein (Mosley *et al.*, 1987). A convertase enzyme that cleaves the IL-1β precursor protein into the active 17 kDa form has been cloned (Cerretti *et al.*, 1993), and efforts to find specific inhibitors are in progress at several pharmaceutical companies.

Blockade of cytokine receptors is another approach to regulating cytokine function. However, efforts to find small organic molecules that directly block receptor binding have generally been unsuccessful. Part of the difficulty is likely a result of the way cytokines bind to their receptors compared to other types of proteins and enzymes. For example, proteolytic enzymes bind and cleave small recognition sequences on target proteins and thus are amenable to inhibition by small molecules that mimic the substrate recognition sequence. Enzymes that act on small molecules such as acetylcholin esterase have relatively small surface areas that interact with those molecules in a specific manner. Since the ligand is small, modifications of ligand structure often produce analogs with the desired agonist or antagonist profile. Cytokines, however, are large polypeptides that interact with their receptors at several points of contact. Thus, mimicking the binding of these proteins to produce antagonists is more complicated. A first approach, generally, is to find small peptide sequences within these protein ligands to successfully compete with the parent protein for receptor binding. Subsequently, synthesis of peptidomimetics is aimed at stabilizing the labile peptide bonds and improving binding affinities. To date, this approach has met with only limited success for cytokine receptors.

Inhibition of inflammatory processes via attenuation of the second messenger signals transduced by ligands binding to their receptors has met with the most success. Xanthine derivatives, for example, have proven to be therapeutically useful presumably by inhibiting phosphodiesterase activity. Studies indicate these compounds suppress the expression levels of TNF-α and IL-1β in myeloid and macrophage cells (Han *et al.*, 1990; Weinberg *et al.*, 1992). Inhibitors of the prostaglandin and leukotriene signalling pathways have also been widely used to reduce inflammatory activity. For example, recently a pilot study using the cyclooxygenase inhibitor indomethacin to treat AD was conducted. Although the trial size and attrition rate were concerns, the results were encouraging enough to proceed with large scale controlled trials (Rogers *et al.*, 1993). Further studies with anti-inflammatory compounds may demonstrate that intervention with the inflammatory and immune-mediated processes is a clinically viable approach, either alone or in conjunction with other treatment regimens.

THE POTENTIAL CONTRIBUTION OF FREE RADICALS TO THE PATHOPHYSIOLOGY OF ALZHEIMER'S DISEASE AND THERAPEUTIC IMPLICATIONS

Oxygen free radicals have been implicated in both the etiology and the post-etiological cascade in many disease states including

AD (Cebellos *et al.*, 1990; Jeandel *et al.*, 1989; Olanow, 1990; Volicer and Crino, 1990). The AD risk factors of aging, brain injury and cerebral ischemia are associated with the production of free radicals (Siesjö *et al.*, 1989; Harman, 1993; Mecocci *et al.*, 1993). Direct evidence for free radical-mediated damage in AD brain is limited to studies demonstrating increased protein oxidation products in frontal cortex (Smith *et al.*, 1991) and increased susceptibility of the temporal and parietal cortices to lipid peroxidation *in vitro* (Subbarao *et al.*, 1990; Hajimohammadreza and Brammer, 1991). Membrane lipid peroxidation may increase the vulnerability of the transmembrane APP to abnormal cleavage by proteases, leading to the deposition of βA4 (Shivers *et al.*, 1988). Altered iron homeostasis may be a contributing factor, since free iron is the most probable agent for lipid peroxidative damage in brain (Arai *et al.*, 1987). Free iron and the regulatory proteins transferrin and ferritin are found around and within senile plaques, microglia and NCT (Jellinger *et al.*, 1990; Connor *et al.*, 1992). Although iron is 67% higher in gray matter in AD brains (Ehmann *et al.*, 1986), the significance of increased levels of iron or aluminium in AD brains has remained controversial (Jellinger *et al.*, 1990; Joshi, 1991; Connor *et al.*, 1992; Evans *et al.*, 1992; Griffiths and Crossman, 1993).

Free radicals may also contribute to conformational changes inducing the formation of both amyloid deposits and paired helical filaments (Ceballos *et al.*, 1988; Dyrks *et al.*, 1988; Shivers *et al.*, 1988; Zemlan *et al.*, 1989; Blass *et al.*, 1990). As described previously, monomeric βA4 can be transformed into aggregating molecules by the addition of metal catalyzed oxidation systems (Dyrks *et al.*, 1992). Possibly by interfering with these oxidative processes, Vitamin E has shown protection of PC12 cells from βA4 toxicity (Behl *et al.*, 1992). Increased activity of glutathione or superoxide dismutase in AD brain, fibroblasts or red blood cells has been interpreted as a conpensatory response to an increased demand for scavenging mechanisms (Zemlan *et al.*, 1989; Adams *et al.*, 1991; Ceballas *et al.*, 1991; Pappolla *et al.*, 1992), however, these findings have not been consistent (Marklund *et al.*, 1985; Perry *et al.*, 1987).

The mechanisms contributing to an increase in free radical production in AD brains are only speculative. Impaired cellular metabolism and mitochondrial function, elevated monoamine oxidase (MAO)-B activity and heavy metal catalyzed oxidation reactions are potential sources. It has been well established that a reduced cerebral metabolic rate for glucose is a predominant abnormality in AD brain (Chase *et al.*, 1983; Cutler *et al.*, 1985; Hoyer *et al.*, 1988, 1992). Compromised cellular energy metabolism and impaired mitochondrial enzyme functions have been postulated to be a consequence of the degeneration of brainstem nuclei, a fundamental aging process accelerated in AD (Hertz, 1989). The loss of noradrenergic neurons (25–90%) in the locus coeruleus and functional noradrenergic deficits are greater in AD than in normal aged individuals (Bondareff *et al.*, 1982; Mann, 1983; Rossor *et al.*, 1984; Marcyniuk *et al.*, 1986; Zweig *et al.*, 1988; Chan-Palay and Asan, 1989). The consequences of a decreased noradrenergic tone include impaired regulation of cerebral blood flow, decreased cellular metabolism of astrocytes, and due to the interdependent relationship of neurons and glia, a depletion of intermediates from the tricarboxylic acid cycle which ultimately compromises neuronal mitochondrial function (Hertz, 1989). In particular, the activities of two enzymes rate-limiting for glucose oxidation, pyruvate dehydrogenase complex and α-ketoglutarate dehydrogenase, are reduced in AD by up to 70% (Sorbi *et al.*, 1983; Sheu *et al.*, 1985; Butterworth and Besnard 1990; Yates *et al.*, 1990; Mastrogiacomo *et al.*, 1993). Deficiencies in mitochondrial cytochrome oxidase and respiratory function may contribute to an increased electron leak and cellular production of free radicals (Sims *et al.*, 1987; Siesjö, 1989; Parker *et al.*, 1990; Kish *et al.*, 1992).

Another potential source of free radicals is MAO-B activity, which generates peroxide in the process of oxidative deamination. MAO-B in increased (10–70%) in AD brain (Reinikainen *et al.*, 1988; Adolfsson *et al.*, 1980; Alexopoulus *et al.*, 1984; Cross *et al.*, 1986; Oreland and Gottfries, 1986; Jossan *et al.*, 1990) and has been localized with reactive astrocytes and senile plaques (Nakamura *et al.*, 1990). The MAO-B inhibitor selegiline (L-deprenyl) has been proposed to have a neuroprotective function based on enhancement of striatal superoxide dismutase activity and prolongation of life span in rats (Knoll, 1992). Long-term DATATOP studes of selegiline in Parkinson's disease, a degenerative disorder affecting the dopaminergic neurons of the substantia nigra, suggest disease-modifying effects by increasing the time required for initiation of L-Dopa therapy, although purely symptomatic effects cannot be ruled out (Parkinson Study Group, 1993). The Alzheimer's Disease Cooperative Study Unit of the National Institutes of Aging is currently studying selegiline for delaying the progression of AD over a two-year period (Hodes, 1994).

Many short term trials with selegiline in AD have been reported (Tariot *et al.*, 1987; Agnoli *et al.*, 1990; Campi *et al.*, 1990; Falsaperla *et al.*, 1990; Monteverde *et al.*, 1990; Piccinin *et al.*, 1990; Finali *et al.*, 1991; Goad *et al.*, 1991; Mangoni *et al.*, 1991; Martignoni *et al.*, 1991; Schneider *et al.*, 1991; Burke *et al.*, 1993. Although cognitive improvements were seen with doses (10 mg/day) below those associated with antidepressant effects (40 mg/day), the data are inconclusive for a disease-modifying effect. Beneficial effects were also reported on the patient's self-adequacy in autonomy of daily living, the management of behavioral problems, anxiety and depression (Monteverde *et al.*, Goad *et al.*, 1991; Mangoni *et al.*, 1991). Thus, the acute cognitive effects may be related to overall improvements in mood and behavior. Additive effects seen with combination treatments of selegiline and cholinesterase inhibitors in pilot studies warrant further investigation (Sunderland *et al.*, 1992; Schneider *et al.*, 1993).

The accumulated evidence suggests that free radical-induced amyloid aggregation and deposition and membrane lipid damage may contribute to the pathophysiology of AD. Thus, interfering with the generation of, or protection from the effects of free radicals may offer therapeutic approaches. The free radical scavengers idebenone and tirilizad mesylate and the iron chelator desferrioxamine have been suggested to be of therapeutic benefit (Crapper-McLachlan, *et al.*, 1991; Hall, 1992; Senin *et al.*, 1992; Nappi *et al.*, 1992), however, clinical trials providing pivotal efficacy data will be required to test this hypothesis.

SUMMARY

This chapter has reviewed some approaches to the development of therapeutics to affect the progression of AD based on our current understanding of several physiological processes which may contribute to the characteristic pathology: APP processing and βA4 generation, cytokine-mediated inflammation and complement activation, and free radical-mediated βA4 aggregation and cellular damage. Several other therapeutic strategies not included here also may have a significant impact on disease progression, e.g. modulation of the phosphorylation state of tau or APP, control of intracellular APP trafficking, interference with CA^{++}-mediated toxicity, and blockers of complement-mediated processes. This list will continue to grow as the etiology of this degenerative disorder is more clearly understood and the fundamental pathological processes to target can be distinguished from secondary events. It is important to note that these approaches propose intervention in the developing AD pathology, as opposed to treatment or reversal of late stage, or fully developed, pathology. An effective treatment therefore depends on reliable diagnostic criteria which correlate to stage of disease progression and early intervention to provide maximal benefit to the patient.

REFERENCES

Abe, K., Tanzi, R. E., and Kogure, K. (1991) Selective induction of kunitz type protease inhibitor domain containing APP mRNA after persistent focal ischaemia in rat cerebral cortex. *Neurosci. Lett.*, **125**, 172–174.

Abraham, C. R., Selkoe, D. J., and Potter, H. (1988) Immunochemical identification of the serine protease inhibitor α_1-antichymotrypsin in the brain amyloid deposits of Alzheimer's disease. *Cell*, **52**, 487–501.

Adams, Jr, J. D., Klaidman, L. K., Odunze, I. N., Shen, H. C., and Miller, C. A. (1991) Alzheimer's and Parkinson's disease: brain levels of glutathione, glutathione disulfide, and vitamin E. *Mol. Chem. Neuropathol.*, **14**, 213–226.

Adolfsson, R., Gottfries, C. G., Oreland, L., Wiberg, A., and Winblad, B. (1980) Increased activity of brain and platelet monoamine oxidase in dementia of Alzheimer type. *Life Sci.*, **27**, 1029–1034.

Agnoli, A., Martucci, N., Fabbrini, G., Buckley, A. E., and Fioravanti, M. (1990) Monoamine oxidase and dementia: Treatment with an inhibitor of MAO-B activity. *Dementia*, **1**, 109–114.

Alexopoulos, G. S., Lieberman, K. W., and Young, R. C. (1984) Platelet MAO activity in primary degenerative dementia. *Am. J. Psychiatry*, **141**, 97–99.

Alsteil, L. D., and Sperber, K. (1991) Cytokines in Alzheimer's disease. *Prog. Neuro-Psychopharmacol. Biol. Psychiatry*, **15**, 481–495.

Anderson, J. P., Esch, F. S., Keim, P. S., Sambamurti, K., Lieberburg, I., and Robakis, N. K. (1991) Exact cleavage site of Alzheimer amyloid precursor in neuronal PC-12 cells. *Neurosci. Lett.*, **128**, 126–128.

Arai, H., Kogure, K., Sugioka, K., and Nakano, M. (1987) Importance of two iron-reducing systems in lipid peroxidation of rat brain: Implications for oxygen toxicity in the central nervous system. *Biochem. Int.*, **14**, 741–749.

Araujo, D. M., and Cotman, C. W. (1992) β-Amyloid stimulates glial cells in vitro to produce growth factors that accumulate in senile plaques in Alzheimer's disease. *Brain Res.*, **569**, 141–145.

Arendt, T., Bigl, B., Tennstedt, A., and Arendt, A. (1984) Correlation between cortical plaque count and neuronal loss in the nucleus basalis in Alzheimer's disease. *Neurosci. Lett.*, **48**, 81–85.

Armstrong, R. A. (1993) Is the clustering of neurofibrillary tangles in Alzheimer's patients related to the cells of origin of specific cortico-cortical projections? *Neurosci. Lett.*, **160**, 57–60.

Ashall, F., and Goate, A. M. (1994) Role of β-amyloid precursor protein in Alzheimer's disease. *Trends Biochem. Sci.*, **19**, 42–46.

Baronti, F., Davis, T. L., Bodry, R. D., Mouradian, M. M., and Chase, T. N. (1992) Deprenyl effects on levodopa pharmacodynamics, mood, and free radical scavenging. *Neurology*, **42**, 541–544.

Bartus, R. T., Dean, R. L., Beer, B., and Lippa, A. S. (1982) The cholinergic hypothesis of geriatric memory dysfunction. *Science*, **217**, 408–417.

Behl, C., Davis, J., Cole, G. M., and Schubert, D. (1992) Vitamin E protects nerve cells from amyloid β protein toxicity. *Biochem. Biophys. Res. Commun.*, **186**, 944–950.

Blass, J. P., Baker, A. C., Ko, L., and Black, R. S. (1990) Induction of Alzheimer antigens by an uncoupler of oxidative phosphorylation. *Arch. Neurol.*, **47**, 864–869.

Bondareff, W., Mountjoy, C. Q., and Roth, M. (1982) Loss of neurons of origin of the adrenergic projection to cerebral cortex (nucleus locus coeruleus) in senile dementia. *Neurology*, **32**, 164–168.

Bowen, D. M. (1988) Neurotransmitters in Alzheimer's disease. *Age*, **11**, 104–110.

Braak, H., and Braak, E. (1991) Neuropathological stageing of Alzheimer-related changes. *Acta Neuropath. (Berl.)*, **82**, 239–259

Bracco, F., Scarpa, M., Rigo, A., and Battistin, L. (1990) Determination of superoxide dismutase activity by the polarographic method of catalytic currents in the cerebrospinal fluid of aging brain and neurologic degenerative diseases. *Proc. Soc. Exp. Biol. Med.*, **196**, 36–41.

Burdick, D., Soreghan, B., Kwon, M., Kosmoski, J., Knauer, M., Henschen, A., Yates, J., Cotman, C., and Glabe, C. (1992) Assembly and aggregation properties of synthetic Alzheimer's A4/β amyloid peptide analogs. *J. Biol. Chem.*, **267**, 546–554.

Burke, W. J., Ranno, A. E., Roccaforte, W. H., Sengel, S. P., Bayer, B. L., and Willcockson, N. K. (1993) L-Deprenyl in the treatment of mild dementia of the Alzheimer type: Preliminary results. *J. Am. Geriatr. Soc.*, 367–370.

Busciglio, J., and Yankner, B. A. (1992) Beta amyloid deposition and neuronal degeneration in cultured human cortical neurons. *Soc. Neurosci. Abs.*, **18**, 1440.

Busciglio, J., Gabuzda, D. H., Matsudaira, P., and Yankner, B. A. (1993) Generation of β-amyloid in the secretory pathway in neuronal and nonneuronal cells. *Proc. Natl Acad. Sci. USA*, **90**, 2092–2096.

Bush, A. I., Pettingell, W. H., Multhaup, G., Paradis, M. D., Vonsattel, J.-P., Gusella, J. F., Beyreuther, K., Masters, C. L., and Tanzi, R. E. (1994) Rapid induction of Alzheimer Aβ amyloid formation by zinc. *Science*, **265**, 1464–1467.

Butterworth, R. F., and Besnard, A.-M. (1990) Thiamine-dependent enzyme changes in temporal cortex of patients with Alzheimer's disease. *Metab. Brain Dis.*, **5**, 179–184.

Buxbaum, J. D., Oishi, M., Chen, H. I., Pinkas-Kramarski, R., Jaffe, E. A., Gandy, S. E., and Greengard, P. (1992) Cholinergic agonists and interleukin-1 regulate processing and secretion of the Alzheimer β/A4 amyloid protein precursor. *Proc. Natl Acad. Sci. USA*, **89**, 10075–10078.

Cai, X-D., Golde, T. E., and Younkin, S. G. (1992) Excess amyloid β protein is released from a mutant amyloid β protein precursor linked to familial Alzheimer's disease. *Science*, **259**, 514–516.

Campi, N., Todeschini, G. P., and Scarzella, L. (1990) Selegiline versus L-acetylcarnitine in the treatment of Alzheimer-type dementia. *Clin. Ther.*, **12**, 306–314.

Caporaso, G. L., Gandy, S. E., Buxbaum, J. D., Ramabhadran, T. V., and Greengard, P. (1992) Protein phosphorylation regulates secretion of Alzheimer β/A4 amyloid precursor protein peptides from β-amyloid precursor protein. *Brain Res.*, **597**, 227–232.

Ceballos, I., Delabar, J. M., Nicole, A., Lynch, R. E., Hallewell, R. A., Kamoun, P., and Sinet, P. M. (1988) Expression of transfected human CuZn superoxide dismutase gene in mouse L cells and NS20Y neuroblastoma cells induces enhancement of glutathione peroxidase activity. *Biochem. Biophys. Acta.*, **949**, 58-64.

Ceballos, I., Javoy-Agid, F., Delacourte, A., Defossez, A., Nicole, A., and Sinet, P. M. (1990) Parkinson's disease and Alzheimer's disease: neurodegenerative disorders due to brain antioxidant system deficiency? *Adv. Exp. Med. Biol.*, **264**, 493–498.

Ceballos, I., Javory-Agic, F., Delacourte, A., Defossez, A., Lafon, M., Hirsch, E., Nicole, A., Sinet, P. M., and Agid, Y. (1991) Neuronal localization of copper–zinc superoxide dismutase protein and mRNA within the human hippocampus from control and Alzheimer's disease brains. *Free Rad. Res. Commun.*, **12–13**, 571–580.

Ceretti, D. P., Koszlosky, C. J., Mosely, B., Nelson, N., VanNess, K., Greenstreet, T. A., March, C. J., Kronheim, S. R., Druck, T., Cannizzaro, L. A., Huebner, K., and Black, R. A. (1993) Molecular cloning of the interleukin-1β converting enzyme. *Science*, **256**, 97–100.

Chan-Palay, V. (1990) Depression and senile dementia of the Alzheimer type: catecholamine changes in the locus coeruleus—Basis for therapy. *Dementia*, **1**, 253–261.

Chan-Palay, V., and Asan, E. (1989) Alterations in catecholamine neurons of the locus coeruleus in senile dementia of the Alzheimer type and in Parkinson's disease with and without dementia and depression. *J. Comp. Neurol.*, **287**, 373–392.

Charmak, B., and Mallat, M. (1991) Fibronectin and laminin regulate the in vitro differentiation of microglial cells. *Neuroscience*, **45**, 513–527.

Chartier-Harlin, M–C., Crawford, M., Houlden, H., Warren, A., Hughes, D., Fidani, L., Goate, A., Rossor, M., Roques, P., Hardy, J., and Mullan, M. (1991) Early-onset Alzheimer's disease caused by mutation at codon 717 of the β-amyloid precursor protein gene. *Nature*, **353**, 844–846.

Chase, T. N., Foster, N. L., Fedio, P., DiChiro, G., Brooks., R., and Patronas, N. (1983) Alzheimer's disease: Local cerebral metabolism studies using the ^{18}F-fluorodeoxy-positron emission tomography technique. In D. Sameule, S. Algeri, S. Gershon, V. E. Grimm, and G. Toffano (eds), *Aging*, vol. 22, *Aging of the Brain*, pp. 143–154, Raven Press, New York.

Citron, M., Oltersdorf, T., Haas, C., McConlogue, L., Hung, A. Y., Seubert, P., Vigo-Pilfrey, C., Lieberburg, I., and Selkoe, D. J. (1992) Mutation of the β-amyloid precursor protein in familial Alzheimer's disease increases β-protein production. *Nature*, **360**, 672–674.

Clemens, J. A., and Stephenson, D. A. (1992) Implants containing β-amyloid protein are not neurotoxic to young and old rat brain. *Neurobiol. Aging*, **13**, 581–586.

Collerton, D. (1986) Cholinergic function and intellectual decline in Alzheimer's disease. *Neuroscience*, **19**, 1–28.

Connor, J. R., Menzies, S. L., St. Martin, S. M., and Mufson, E. J. (1992) A histochemical study of iron, transferrin, and ferritin in Alzheimer's disease brains. *J. Neurosci. Res.*, **31**, 75–83.

Corder, E. H., Saunders, A. M., Strittmatter, W. J., Schmechel, D. E., Gaskell, P. C., Small, G. W., Roses, A. D., Haines, J. L., and Patrick-Vance, M. A. (1993) Gene dose of apolipoprotein E type 4 allele and the risk of Alzheimer's disease in late onset families. *Science*, **261**, 921–923.

Crapper-McLachlan, D. R., Dalton, A. J., Kruck, T. P. A., Bell, M. Y., Smith, W. L., Kalow, W., and Andrews, D. F. (1991) Intramuscular desferrioxamine in patients with Alzheimer's disease. *Lancet*, **337**, 1304–1308.

Cras, P., Kawai, M., Siedlak, S., Mulvihill, P., Ganbetti, P., Lowey, D., Gonzalez-DeWhitt, P., Greenberg, P., and Perry, G. (1990) Neuronal and microglial involvement in β-amyloid protein deposition in Alzheimer's disease. *Am. J. Pathol.*, **137**, 241–246.

Cras, P., Kawai, M., Siedlak, S., and Perry, G. (1991) Microglia are associated with the extracellular neurofibillary tangles of Alzheimer's disease. *Brain Res.*, **558**, 312–314.

Cross, A. J., Crow, T. J., Dawson, J. M., Ferrier, I. N., Johnson, J. A., Peter, T. J., and Reynolds, G. P. (1986) Subcellular pathology of human neurodegenerative disorders: Alzheimer-type dementia and Huntington's disease. *J. Neurochem.*, **47**, 882–889.

Crowther, R. A., Oleson, O. F., Jakes, R., and Goedert, M. (1992) The microtubule binding repeats of tau protein assemble into filaments like those found in Alzheimer's disease. *FEBS Lett.*, **309**, 199–202.

Cutler, N. R., Haxby, J. V., Duara, R., Grady, C. L., Kay, A. D., Kessler, R.M., Sundaram, M., and Rapoport, S. I. (1985) Clinical history, brain metabolism, and neuropsychological function in Alzheimer's disease. *Ann. Neurol.*, **18**, 298–309.

Davis, K. L., Thal, L. J., Gamzu, E. R., Davis, C.W., Woolson, R. F., Gracon, S. I., Drachman, D. A., Schneider, L. S., Whitehouse, P. J., Hoover, T. M., Morris, J. C., Kawas, C. H., Knopman, D. S., Earl, N. L., Kumar, V., and Doody, R. S. (1992) A double-blind, placebo-controlled multicenter study of tacrine for Alzheimer's disease. *N. Engl. J. Med.*, **327**, 1253–1259.

DeLacoste, M.-C., and White, C. L., III (1993) The role of cortical connectivity in Alzheimer's disease pathogenesis; a review and model system. *Neurobiol. Aging*, **14**, 1–16.

Delacourte, A., Defossez, A., Ceballos, I., Nicole, A., and Sinet, P. M. (1988) Preferential localization of copper zinc superoxide dismutase in the vulnerable cortical neurons in Alzheimer's disease. *Neurosci. Lett.*, **92**, 247–253.

Dickson, D. W., Farlo, J., Davies, P., Crystal, H., Fuld, P., and Yen, S-H. C. (1988) A double-labeling immunohistochemical study of senile plaques. *Am. J. Pathol.*, **132**, 86–101.

Donnelly, R. J., Friedhoff, A. J., Beer, B., Blum, A. J., and Viṭek, M. P. (1990) Interleukin-1 stimulates the beta-amyloid precursor protein promoter. *Cell. Mol. Neurobiol.*, **10**, 485–495.

Dyrks, T., Weidemann, A., Multhaup, G., Salbaum, J. M., Lemaire, H.–G., Kang, J., Müller-Hill, B., Masters, C. L., and Beyreuther, K. (1988) Identification, transmembrane orientation and biogenesis of the amyloid A4 precursor of Alzheimer's disease. *EMBO J.*, **7**, 949–957.

Dyrks, T., Dyrks, E., Hartman, T., Masters, C. L., and Beyreuther, K. (1992) Amyloidogenicity of βA4 and βA4-bearing amyloid protein precursor fragments by metal-catalyzed oxidation. *J. Biol. Chem.*, **267**, 18210–18217.

Dyrks, T., Dyrks, E., Masters, C. L., and Beyreuther, K. (1993) Amyloidogenicity of rodent and human βA4 sequences. *FEBS Lett.*, **324**, 231–236.

Ehmann, W. D., Markesberry, W. R., Alauddin, M., Hussain, T. I. M., and Brubak, E. H. (1986) Brain trace elements in Alzheimer's disease. *Neurotoxicol.*, **7**, 197–206.

Eikelenboom, P., and Stam, F. C. (1982) Immunoglobulins and complement factors in senile plaques. *Acta Neuropathol (Berl.)*, **57**, 239–242.

Emre, M. C., Geula, C., Ransil, B. J., and Mesulam, M. M. (1992) The acute neurotoxicity and effects upon cholinergic axons of intracerebrally injected β-amyloid in the rat brain. *Neurobiol. Aging*, **13**, 553–560.

Esch, F. S., Keim, P. S., Beattie, E. C., Blacher, R. W., Culwell, A. R., Oltersdorf, T., McClure, D., and Ward, P. J. (1990) Cleavage of amyloid β-peptide during constitutive processing of its precursor. *Science*, **248**, 112–1124.

Evans, P. H., Pethans, E., Burge, T., and Klinowski, L. J. (1992) Aluminosilicate-induced free radical generation by murine brain glial cells in vitro: potential significance in the aetiopathogenesis of Alzheimer's dementia. *Dementia*, **3**, 1–6.

Falsaperla, A., Pretti, P. A. M., and Oliani, C. (1990) Selegiline versus oxiracetam in patients with Alzheimer-type dementia. *Clin. Ther.*, **12**, 315–322.

Farlow, M., Gracon, S. I., Hershey, L. A., Lewis, K. W., Sadowsky, C. H., Dolan-Ureno, J. for the Tacrine Study Group (1992) A controlled trial of tacrine in Alzheimer's disease. *JAMA*, **268**, 2525–2532.

Fibiger, H. C. (1991) Cholinergic mechanisms in learning, memory and dementia: A review of recent evidence. *Trends Neurosci.*, **14**, 220–223.

Finali, G., Piccirilli, M., Oliani, C., *et al.* (1991) L-Deprenyl therapy improves verbal memory in amnesic Alzheimer patients. *Clin. Neuropharmacol.*, **14**, 523–536.

Frautschy, S. A., Baird, A., and Cole, G. M. (1991) Effects of injected Alzheimer β-amyloid cores in rat brain. *Proc. Natl Acad. Sci. USA*, **88**, 8362–8366.

Frautschy, S. A., Cole, G. M., and Baird, A. (1992) Phagocytosis and deposition of vascular β-amyloid in rat brains injected with Alzheimer β-amyloid. *Am. J. Pathol.*, **140**, 1389–1399.

Games, D., Khan, K. M., Sorinao, F. G., Davis, D. L., Bryant, K., and Lieberburg, I. (1992) Lack of Alzheimer pathology after β-amyloid protein injections in rat brain. *Neurobiol. Aging*, **13**, 569–576.

Ganter, U., Strauss, S., Jonal, U., Weidemann, A., Beyreuther, K., Volk, B., Berger, M., and Bauer, J. (1991) Alpha-2-macroglobulin synthesis in interleukin-6-stimulated human neuronal (SH-SY5Y) neuroblastoma cells: potential significance for the processing of Alzheimer β-amyloid precursor protein. *FEBS Lett.*, **282**, 127–131.

Gentleman, S. M., Nash, M. J., Sweeting, C. J., Graham, D. I., and Roberts, G. W. (1993) β-Amyloid precursor protein (βAPP) as a marker for axonal injury after head injury. *Neurosci. Lett.*, **160**, 139–144.

Glenner, G., and Wong, C. (1984) Alzheimer's disease: initial report of the purification and characterization of a novel cerebrovascular amyloid protein. *Biochem. Biophys. Res. Commun.*, **120**, 885–890.

Goad, D. L., Davis, C. M., Liem, P., Fuselier, C. C., McCormack, J. R., and Olsen, K. M. (1991) The use of selegiline in Alzheimer's patients with behavior problems. *J. Clin. Psychiatry*, **42**, 342–345.

Goate, A., Chartie-Harlin, M. C., Mullan, M., Brown, J., Crawford, F., Fidani, L., Giuffra, L., Haynes, A., Irving, N., James, L., Mant, R., Newton, P., Rook, K., Roques, P., Talbot, C., Pericak-Vance, M., Roses, A., Williamson, R., Rossen, M., Owen, M., and Hardy, J. (1991) Segregation of a missense mutation in the amyloid precursor protein gene with familial Alzheimer's disease. *Nature*, **349**, 704–706.

Goedert, M. (1993) Tau protein and the neurofibrillary pathology of Alzheimer's disease. *Trends Neurosci.*, **16**, 460–465.

Goedert, M., Cohen, E. S., Jakes, R., and Cohen, P. (1992) p42MAP kinase phosphorylation sites in microtubule-associated protein tau are dephosphorylated by protein phosphatase 2A1. *FEBS Lett.*, **312**, 95–99.

Goedert, M., Spillantini, M. G., Cairns, N. J., and Crowther, R. A. (1992) Tau proteins of Alzheimer paired helical filaments: abnormal phosphorylation of all six brain isoforms. *Neuron*, **8**, 159–168.

Golde, T. E., Estus, S., Usiak, M., Younkin, L. H., and Younkin, S. G. (1990) Expression of the amyloid protein precursor mRNAs: recognition of a novel alternatively spliced form and quantitation in Alzheimer's disease using PCR. *Neuron*, **4**, 253–267.

Goldgaber, D., Lerman, M. J., McBride, O. W., Saffiotti, U., and Gajdusek, D. C. (1987) Characterization and chromosomal localization of a cDNA encoding brain amyloid of Alzheimer's disease. *Science*, **235**, 877–880.

Goldgaber, M. D., Harris, H., Hla, T., Maciag, T., Donnelly, R. J., Jacobsen, J. S. Vitek, M. P., and Gajdusek, D. C. (1989) Interleukin-1 regulates synthesis of amyloid β-protein precursor mRNA in human endothelial cells. *Proc. Natl Acad. Sci. USA*, **86**, 7606–7610.

Gottfries, C. G. (1985) Alzheimer's disease and senile dementia: biochemical characteristics and aspects of treatment. *Psychopharmacology*, **86**, 245–252.

Graves, A. B., White, E., Koepsell, T. D., Reifler, B. V., van Belle, G., Larson, E. B., and Raskind, M. (1990) The association between head trauma and Alzheimer's disease. *Am. J. Epidemiol.*, **131**, 491–501.

Griffen, W. S. T., Stanley, L. C., Ling, C., White, L., MacLeod, V., Perrot, L. F., White III, C. L., and Araoz, C. (1989) Brain interleukin 1 and S-100 immunoreactivity are elevated in Down syndrome and Alzheimer disease. *Proc. Natl Acad. Sci. USA*, **86**, 7611–7615.

Griffiths, P. D. and Crossman, A. R. (1993) Distribution of iron in the basal ganglia and neocortex in postmortem tissue in Parkinson's disease and Alzheimer's disease. *Dementia*, **4**, 61–65.

Haass, C., Koo, E. H., Mellon, A., Hung, A. Y., and Selkoe, D. J. (1992a) Targeting of cell-surface β-amyloid precursor protein to lysosomes: alternative processing into amyloid bearing fragments. *Nature*, **357**, 500–503.

Haass, C., Schlossmacher, M. G., Hung, A. Y., Vigo-Pilfrey, C., Mellon, A., Ostaszweski, B. L., Lieberburg, I., Koo, E. H., Schenk, D., Teplow, D. B., and Selkoe, D. J. (1992b) Amyloid β-peptide is produced by cultured cells during normal metabolism. *Nature*, 359, 325–327.

Haga, S., Akai, K., and Ishii, T. (1989) Demonstration of microglial cells in and around senile (neuritic) plaques in the Alzheimer brain. *Acta Neuropathol. (Berl.)*, **77**, 569–575.

Haga, S., Ikeda, K., Sato, M., and Ishii, T. (1993) Synthetic Alzheimer amyloid β/A4 peptides enhance production of complement C3 component by cultured microglial cells. *Brain Res.*, **601**, 88–94.

Hajimohammadreza, I., and Brammer, M. (1991) Brain membrane fluidity and lipid peroxidation in Alzheimer's disease. *Neurosci. Lett.*, **112**, 333–337.

Hall, E. D. (1992) Novel inhibitors of iron-dependent lipid peroxidation for neurogenerative disorders. *Ann. Neurol.*, **32**, Suppl, S-137–142.

Han, J., Thompson, P., and Beutler, B. (1990) Dexamethasone and pentoxyfylline inhibit endotoxin-induced cachectin/tumor necrosis factor synthesis at separate points in the signaling pathway. *J. Exp. Med.*, **172**, 391–394.

Hardy, J. A., and Higgins, G. A. (1992) Alzheimer's disease: the amyloid cascade hypothesis. *Science*, **256**, 184–185.

Harman, D. (1993) Free radical theory of aging: A hypothesis on pathogenesis of senile dementia of the Alzheimer type. *Age*, **16**, 23–30.

Henderson, A. S. (1988) The risk factors for Alzheimer's disease: A review and a hypothesis. *Acta Psychiatr. Scand.*, **78**, 257–275.

Hertz, L. (1989) Is Alzheimer's disease an anterograde degeneration, originating in the brainstem, and disrupting metabolic and functional interactions between neurons and glial cells? *Brain Res. Rev.*, **14**, 335–353.

Hodes, R. J. (1944) Alzheimer's disease: Treatment research finds new targets. *J. Am. Geriatr. Soc.*, **42**, 679–681.

Holttum, J. R., and Gershon, S. (1992) The cholinergic model of dementia, Alzheimer type: progression from the unitary transmitter concept. *Dementia*, **3**, 174–185.

Hoyer, S. (1992) Oxidative energy metabolism in Alzheimer brain. Studies in early-onset and late-onset cases. *Mol. Chem. Neuropathol.*, **16**, 207–224.

Hoyer, S., Oesterreich, K., and Wagner, O. (1988) Glucose metabolism as the site of the primary abnormality in early-onset dementia of Alzheimer type? *J. Neurol.*, **235**, 143–148.

Hyman, B. T., Marzloff, K., and Arriagada, P. V. (1993) The lack of accumulation of senile plaques or amyloid burden in Alzheimer's disease suggests a dynamic balance between amyloid deposition and resolution. *J. Neuropathol. Exp. Neurol.*, **52**(6), 594–600.

Jarrett, J. T., and Lansbury, Jr, P. T. (1993) Seeding 'one dimensional crystallization' of amyloid: A pathogenic mechanism in Alzheimer's disease and scrapie? *Cell*, **73**, 1055–1058.

Jarrett, J. T., Berger, E. P., and Lansbury, Jr, P. T. (1993) The carboxy-terminus of the β amyloid protein is critical for the seeding of amyloid formation: implications for the pathogenesis of Alzheimer's disease. *Biochemistry*, **32**, 4693–4697.

Jeandel, C., Nicolas, M. B., Dubois, F., Nabet-Belleville, F., Penin, F., and Cuny, G. (1989) Lipid peroxidation and free radical scavengers in Alzheimer's disease. *Gerontology*, **35**, 275–282.

Jellinger, K., Paulus, W., Grundke-Iqbal, I., Riderer, P., and Youdim, M. B. H. (1990) Brain iron and ferritin in Parkinson's and Alzheimer's diseases. *J. Neuronal Transm. (P–D Sect.)*, **2**, 327–340.

Jones, J. T., Morris, S., Yates, C. M., Moffoot, A., Sharpe, C., Brock, D. J. H., and St. Clair, D. (1992) Mutation in codon 713 of the β-amyloid precursor protein gene presenting with schizophrenia. *Nature Genet.*, **1**, 306–309.

Joshi, J. G. (1991) Neurochemical hypothesis: participation by aluminium in producing critical mass of colocalized errors in brain leads to neurological disease. *Comp. Biochem. Physiol.*, **100C**, 103–105.

Jossan, S. S., Gillberg, P. G., Karlsson, I., Gottfries, C. G., and Oreland, L. (1990) Visualization of brain monoamine oxidase B (MAO-B) in dementia of Alzheimer's type by means of large crysection autoradiography: a pilot study. *J. Neural. Transm.*, **325**, 61-5.

Jossan, S. S., Gillberg, P. G., Gottfries, C. G., Karlsson, I., and Oreland, L. (1991) Monamine oxidase B in brains from patients with Alzheimer's disease: a biochemical and autoradiographical study. *Neuroscience.*, **45**, 1–12.

Kang, J., Lemaire, H. G., Unterbeck, A., Salbaum, J. M., Masters, C. L., Grzeschik, K. H., Malthaup, G., Beyreuther, K., and Muller-Hill, B. (1987) The precursor of Alzheimer's disease amyloid A4 protein resembles cell surface receptor. *Nature*, **325**, 733–736.

Katzman, R. and Saitoh, T. (1991) Advances in Alzheimer's disease. *FASEB J.*, **5**, 278–286.

Kawarabayashi, T., Shoji, M., Harigaya, Y., Yamaguchi, H., and Hirai, S. (1991) Expression of APP in the early stage of brain damage. *Brain Res.*, **563**, 334–338.

Kimura, H., and Schubert, D. (1993) Amyloid β-protein activates tachykinin receptors and inositol trisphosphate accumulation by synergy with glutamate. *Proc. Natl Acad. Sci. USA*, **90**, 7508–7512.

Kish, S. J., Bergeron, C., Rajput, A., Dozic, S., Mastrogiacomo, F., Chang, L.-J., Wilson, J. M., DiStefano, L. M., and Nobrega, J. N. (1992)

Cytochrome oxidase in Alzheimer's disease. *J. Neurochem.*, **59**, 776–779.

Kitaguchi, N., Takahashi, Y., Tokushima, Y., Shiojiri, S., Ito, H. (1988) Novel precursor of Alzheimer's disease amyloid protein shows protease inhibitory activity. *Nature*, **331**, 530–532

Knauer, M. F., Soreghan, B., Burdick, D., Kosmoski, J., and Glabe, C. G. (1992) Intracellular accumulation and resistance to degradation of the Alzheimer's amyloid A4/β protein. *Proc. Natl Acad. Sci. USA*, **89**, 7437–7441.

Knoll, J. (1992) Pharmacological basis of the therapeutic effect of (-)deprenyl in age-related neurological diseases. *Med. Res. Rev.*, **12**, 505–524.

Konig, G., Monning, U., Czech, C., Prior, R., Banati, R., Schreiter-Gasser, U., Bauer, J., Masters, C. L., and Beyreuther, K. (1992) Identification and differential expression of a novel alternative splice isoform of the βA4 amyloid precursor protein (APP) mRNA in leukocytes and brain microglial cells. *J. Biol. Chem.*, **267**, 10804–10809.

Kosik, K. S. (1992) Alzheimer's disease: a cell biological perspective. *Science*, **256**, 780–783.

Kowall, N. W., McKee, A. C., Yankner, B. A., and Beal, M. F. (1991) An in vivo model for the neurodegenerative effects of β amyloid and protection by substance P. *Proc. Natl Acad. Sci. USA*, **88**, 7247–7251.

Kowall, N. W., McKee, A. C., Yankner, B. A., and Beal, M. F. (1992) In vivo neurotoxicity of beta amyloid [β (1–40)] and the [β (25–35)] fragment. *Neurobiol. Aging*, **13**, 537–542.

Lees, G. J. (1993) Contributory mechanisms in the causation of neurodegenerative disorders. *Neuroscience*, **54**, 287–322.

Loo, D. T., Copani, A., Pike, C. J., Whittemore, E. R., Walencewicz, A. J., and Cotman, C. W. (1993) Apoptosis is induced by β-amyloid in cultured central nervous system neurons. *Proc. Natl Acad. Sci. USA*, **90**, 7951–7955.

Lue, L.-F., and Rogers, J. (1992) Full complement activation fails in diffuse plaques of the Alzheimer's disease cerebellum. *Dementia*, **3**, 308–313.

Mangoni, A., Grassi, M. P., Frattola, L., Piolti, R., Bassi, S., Motta, A., Marcone, A., and Smirne, S. (1991) Effects of a MAO-B inhibitor in the treatment of Alzheimer disease. *Eur. Neurol.*, **31**, 100–107.

Mann, D. M. (1983) The locus coeruleus and its possible role in ageing and degenerative disease of the human central nervous system. *Mech. Ageing Dev.*, **23**, 73–94.

Mann, D. M., Yates, P. O., and Marcyniuk, B. (1985) Correlation between senile plaque and neurofibrillary tangle counts in cerebral cortex and neuronal counts in cortex and subcortical structures in Alzheimer's disease. *Neurosci. Lett.*, **56**, 51–55.

Marcyniuk, B., Mann, D. M., and Yates, P. O. (1986) The topography of cell loss from locus coeruleus in Alzheimer's disease. *J. Neurol. Sci.*, **76**, 335–45.

Marklund, S. L., Adolfsson, R., Gottfries, C. G., and Winblad, B. (1985) Superoxide dismutase isoenzymes in normal brains and in brains from patients with dementia of Alzheimer type. *J. Neurol. Sci.*, **67**, 319–325.

Martignoni, E., Bono, G., Blandini, F., Sinforiani, E., Merlo, P., and Nappi, G. (1991) Monamines and related metabolite levels in the cerebrospinal fluid of patients with dementia of Alzheimer's type. Influence of treatment with L-deprenyl. *J. Neural. Transm. (P–D Sect.)*, **3**, 15–25.

Maruyama, K., Usami, M., Yamao-Harigaya, W., Tagawa, K., and Ishiura, S. (1991) Mutation of Glu-693 or Val-717 to Ile has no effect on the processing of Alzheimer amyloid precursor protein expressed in cos-1 cells by cDNA transfection. *Neurosci. Lett.*, **132**, 97–100.

Masters, C., Multhaup, G., Simms, G., Pottgeisser, J., Martins, R., and Beyreuther, K. (1985a) Neuronal origin of a cerebral amyloid: neurofibrillary tangles of Alzheimer's disease contain the same protein as the amyloid of plaque cores and blood vessels. *EMBO J.*, **4**, 2757–2763.

Masters, C. L., Simms, G., Weinmann, N. A., Multhaup, G., McDonald, B. L., and Beyreuther, K. (1985b) Amyloid plaque core protein in Alzheimer's disease and Down's syndrome. *Proc. Natl Acad. Sci. USA*, **82**, 4245–4249.

Mastrogiacomo, F., Bergeron, C., and Kish, S. J. (1993) Brain α-ketoglutarate dehydrogenase complex activity in Alzheimer's disease. *J. Neurochem.*, **61**, 2007–2014.

Mattson, M. P., Cheng, B., Davis, D., Bryant, K., Lieberburg, I., and Rydel, R. E. (1992) β-amyloid peptides destabilize calcium homeostasis and render human cortical neurons vulnerable to excitotoxicity. *J. Neurosci.*, **12**, 376–389.

Mattson, M. P., Barger, S. W., Cheng, B., Lieberburg, I., Smith-Swintosky, V. L., and Rydel, R. E. (1993) β-Amyloid precursor protein metabolites and loss of neuronal Ca^{2+} homeostasis in Alzheimer's disease. *Trends Neurosci.*, **16**, 409–414.

May, P. C., Gitter, B. D., Waters, D.C., Simmons, L. K., Becker, G. W., Small, J. S., and Robison, P. M. (1992) β-amyloid peptide in vitro toxicity: lot-to-lot variability. *Neurobiol. Aging*, **13**, 605–608.

McGeer, P. L., and Rogers, J. (1992) Anti-inflammatory agents as a therapeutic approach to Alzheimer's disease. *Neurology*, **42**, 447–449.

McGeer, P. L., Itagaki, S., Tago, H., and McGeer, E. G. (1987) Reactive microglia in patients with senile dementia of the Alzheimer type are positive for the histocompatibility of glycoprotein HLA-DR. *Neurosci. Lett.*, **79**, 195–200.

McGeer, P. L., Itagaki, S., Boyes, B. E., and McGeer, E. G. (1988) Reactive microglia are positive for HLA-DR in the substantia nigra of Parkinson's and Alzheimer's disease brains. *Neurology.*, **38**, 1285–1291.

McGeer, P. L., Akiyama, H., Itagaki, S., and McGeer, E. G. (1989) Immune system response in Alzheimer's disease. *Can. J. Neurol. Sci.*, **16**, 516–527.

McGeer, P. L., Walker, D. G., Akiyama, H., Kawamata, T., Guan, A. L., Parker, C. J., Okada, N., and McGeer, E. G. (1991) Detection of the membrane inhibitor of reactive lysis (CD59) in diseased neurons of Alzheimer brain. *Brain Res.*, **544**, 315–319.

McGeer, P. L., Haruda, N., Kimura, H., McGeer, E. G., and Schulzer, M. (1992) Prevalence of dementia amongst elderly Japanese with leprosy: apparent effect of chronic drug therapy. *Dementia*, **3**, 146–149.

Mecocci, P., MacGarvey, U., Kaufman, A. E., Koontz, D., Shoffner, J. M., Wallace, D. C., and Beal, M. F. (1993) Oxidative damage to mitochondrial DNA shows marked age-dependent increases in human brain. *Ann. Neurol.*, **34**, 609–616.

Miller, D. L., Papayannopoulus, I. A., Styles, J., Bobin, S. A., Lin, Y. Y., Biemann, K., and Iqbal, K. (1992a) Peptide compositions of the cerebrovascular and senile plaque core amyloid deposits of Alzheimer's Disease. *Arch. Biochem. Biophys.*, **301**, 41–52.

Miller, S. W., Mahoney, J. M., and Jann, M. W. (1992b) Therapeutic frontiers in Alzheimer's disease. *Pharmacotherapy*, **12**, 217–231.

Monteverde, A., Gnemmi, P., Rossi, F., and Monteverde, A. (1990) Selegiline in the treatment of mild to moderate Alzheimer-type dementia. *Clin. Ther.*, **12**, 315–322.

Mosley, B., Urdal, D., Prickett, K., Larsen, A., Cosman, D., Conlon, P., Gillis, S., and Dower, S. K. (1987) The interleukin-1 receptor binds the human interleukin-1α precursor but not the interleukin-1β precursor. *J. Biol. Chem.*, **262**, 2941–2944.

Mullan, M., Crawford, F., Axelman, K., Houlden, H., Lilius, L., Winbald, B., and Lannfelt, L. (1992) A pathogenic mutation for probable Alzheimer's disease in the APP gene at the N-terminus of β-amyloid. *Nature Genet.*, **1**, 345–347.

Murrell, J., Farlow, M., Ghetti, B., and Benson, M. D. (1991) A mutation in amyloid precursor protein associated with hereditary Alzheimer's disease. *Science*, **254**, 97–99.

Nakajima, K., and Kohsaka, S. (1993) Functional roles of microglia in the brain. *Neurosci. Res.*, **17**, 187–203.

Nakamura, S., Kawamata, T., Akiguchi, I., Kameyama, M., Nakamura, N., and Kimura, H. (1990) Expression of monoamine oxidase-B activity in astrocytes of senile plaques. *Acta Neuropathol.*, **80**, 419–425.

Nappi, G., Bono, G., Merlo, P., Denaro, A., Proietti, R., Martocci, N., and Fiorauanti, M. (1992) Long-term idebenone treatment of vascular and degenerative brain disorders of the elderly. *Arch. Gerontol. Geriatr.*, **15**, 261–269.

Nitsch, R. M., Slack, B. E., Wurtman, R. J., and Growdon, J. H. (1992) Release of Alzheimer amyloid precursor derivatives stimulated by activation of muscarinic acetylcholine receptors. *Science*, **258**, 304–307.

Olanow, C. W. (1990) Oxidation reactions in Parkinson's disease. *Neurology*, **40** (Suppl. 3, No. 10), 32–39.

Oltersdorf, T., Ward, P., Henriksson, T., Beattie, E. C., Neve, R., Lieberburg, I., and Fritz, L. C. (1990) The Alzheimer's amyloid protein: identification of a stable intermediate in the biosynthetic/degradative pathway. *J. Biol. Chem.*, **265**, 4492–4497.

Oreland, L., and Gottfries, C. G. (1986) Brain and brain monamine oxidase in aging and in dementia of Alzheimer's type. *Prog. Neuro-Psychopharmacol. Biol. Psychiatry*, **10**, 533–540.

Palmer, A. M., and Gershon, S. (1990) Is the neuronal basis of Alzheimer's disease cholinergic or glutamatergic? *FASEB J.*, **4**, 2745–2752.

Pappolla, M. A., Omar, R. A., Kim, K. S., and Robakis, N. K. (1992) Immunohistochemical evidence of antioxidant stress in Alzheimer's disease. *Am. J. Pathol.*, **140**, 621–628.

Parker, W. D., Filley, C. F., and Parks, J. K. (1990) Cytochrome oxidase deficiency in Alzheimer's disease. *Neurology*, **40**, 1302–1303.

Parkinson Study Group (1993) Effects of tocopherol and deprenyl on the progression of disability in early Parkinson's disease. *N. Engl. J. Med.*, **328**, 176–183.

Pearson, R. C. A., Esiri, M. M., Hiorns, R. W., Wilcock, G. K., and Powel, T. P. S. (1985) Anatomical correlates of the distribution of the pathological changes in the neocortex of Alzheimer's disease. *Proc. Natl Acad. Sci. USA*, **82**, 4531–4534.

Perlmutter, L. S., Barron, E., and Chui, H. C. (1990) Morphologic association between the microglia and senile plaque amyloid in Alzheimer's disease. *Neurosci. Lett.*, **119**, 32–36.

Perlmutter, L. S., Scott, S. A., Barron, E., and Chui, H. C. (1992) MHC Class II-positive microglia in human brain: association with Alzheimer lesions. *J. Neurosci. Res.*, **33**, 549–558.

Perrin, R., Briancon, S., Jeandel, C., Artur, Y., Minn, A., Penin, F., and Siest, G. (1990) Blood activity of Cu/Zn superoxide dismutase, glutathione peroxidase and catalase in Alzheimer's disease: a case–control study. *Gerontology*, **36**, 306–313.

Perry, T. L., Yong, V. W., Bergeron, C., Hansen, S., and Jones, K. (1987) Amino acids, glutathione, and glutathione transferase activity in the brains of patients with Alzheimer's disease. *Ann. Neurol.*, **21**, 331–336.

Perry, V. P., Andersson, P.–B., and Gordon, S. (1993) Macrophages and inflammation in the central nervous system. *Trends Neurosci.*, **16**, 268–273.

Piccinin, G.L., Finali, G., and Piccirilli, M. (1990) Neuropsychological effects of L-deprenyl in Alzheimer's type dementia. *Clin. Neuropharmacol.*, **13**, 147–163.

Pike, C. J., Walencewicz, A. J., Glabe, C. G., and Cotman, C. W. (1991) In vitro aging of β-amyloid protein causes peptide aggregation and neurotoxicity. *Brain Res.*, **563**, 311–314.

Pike, C. J., Burdick, D., Walencewicz, A. J., Glabe, C. G., and Cotman, C. W. (1993) Neurodegeneration induced by β-amyloid peptides in vitro: the role of peptide assembly state. *J. Neurosci.*, **13**, 1676–1687.

Podlinsky, M. B., Stephenson, D. T., Frosch, M. P., Lieberburg, I., Clemens, J. A., and Selkoe, D. J. (1992) Synthetic amyloid β-protein fails to produce specific neurotoxicity in monkey cerebral cortex. *Neurobiol. Aging*, **13**, 561–568.

Rebec, G. W., Reiter, J. S., Strickland, D. K., and Hyman, B. T. (1993) Apolipoprotein E in sporadic Alzheimer's disease: allelic variation and receptor interactions. *Neuron*, **11**, 575–580.

Refolo, L. M., Salton, S. R. J., Anderson, J. P., Mehta, P., and Robakis, N. K. (1989) Nerve and epidermal growth factors induce the release of the Alzheimer amyloid precursor from PC-12 cell cultures. *Biochem. Biophys. Res. Commun.*, **164**, 664–670.

Reinikainen, K. J., Paljarvi, L., Halonen, T., Maloninen, O., Kosam, V.-M., Laakso, M., and Rickkinen, P. J. (1988) Dopaminergic systems and monamine oxidase-B activity in Alzheimer's disease. *Neurobiol. Aging*, **9**, 2545–2552.

Robakis, N. K., Wisniewski, H. M., Jenkins, E. C., Devin-Gage, E. A., Houck, G. E., Yao, X-L., Ramakrishna, N., Wolfe, G., Silverman, W. P., and Brown, W. T. (1987) Chromosome 21q21 sublocalization of a gene encoding β-amyloid peptide in cerebral vessels and neuritic (senile) plaques of people with Alzheimer's disease and Down's syndrome. *Lancet*, **i**, 384–385.

Rogers, J., Civin, W. H., Styren, S. D., and McGeer, P. L. (1992a) Immune-related mechanisms of Alzheimer's disease pathogenesis, in Z. S. Khachaturian and J. P. Blass (eds), *Alzheimer's Disease, New Treatment Strategies.* Marcel Dekker, New York, pp. 147–162.

Rogers, J., Cooper, N. R., Webster, S., Schultz, J., McGeer, P. L., Styren, S. D., Civin, W. H., Brachova, L., Bradt, B., Ward, P., and Lieberburg, I. (1992b) Complement activation by β-amyloid in Alzheimer disease. *Proc. Natl Acad. Sci. USA*, **89**, 10016–10020.

Rogers, J., Kirby, L. C., Hempelman, S. R., Berry, D. L., McGeer, P. L., Kaszniak, A. W., Zalinski, J., Cofield, M., Mansukhani, L., Willson, P., and Kogan, F. (1993) Clinical trial of indomethacin in Alzheimer's disease. *Neurology*, **43**, 1609–1611.

Rossor, M. N., Iverson, L. L., Reynolds, G. P., and Mountjoy, C. Q. (1984) Neurochemical characteristics of early and late onset type of Alzheimer's disease. *Br. Med. J.*, **288**, 961–964.

Rozemuller, J. M., Eikelenboom, P., Stam, F. C., Beyreuther, K., and Masters, C. L. (1989) A4 protein in Alzheimer's disease: primary and secondary cellular events in extracellular amyloid deposition. *J. Neuropathol. Exp. Neurol.*, **48**, 674–691.

Rush, D. K., Aschimies, S., and Merriman, M. C. (1992) Intracerebral β-amyloid (25–35) produces tissue damage. Is it neurotoxic? *Neurobiol. Aging*, **13**, 591–594.

Sahasrabudhe, S. R., Spruyt, M. A., Muenkel, M. A., Blume, A. J., Vitek, M. P., and Jacobsen, J. S. (1992) Release of amino-terminal fragments from amyloid precursor protein reporter and mutated derivatives in cultured cells. *J. Biol. Chem.*, **267**, 25602–25608.

Sambamurti, K., Shioi, J., Anderson, J. P., Pappolla, M. A., and Robakis, N. K. (1992) Evidence for intracellular cleavage of the Alzheimer's amyloid precursor in PC12 cells. *J. Neurosci. Res.*, **33**, 319–329.

Schneider, L. S., Pollock, V. E., Zemansky, M. F., Gleason, R. P., Palmer, R., and Sloane, B. (1991) A pilot study of low-dose L-deprenyl in Alzheimer's disease. *J. Geriatr. Psychiatry Neurol.*, **4**, 143–148.

Schneider, L. S., Olin, J. T., and Pawluczyk, S. (1993) A double-blind crossover pilot study of L-deprenyl (selegiline) combined with cholinesterase inhibitor in Alzheimer's disease. *Am. J. Psychiatry*, **150**, 321–323.

Selkoe, D. J. (1991) The molecular pathology of Alzheimer's disease. *Neuron*, **6**, 487–498.

Selkoe, D. J. (1993) Physiological production of the β-amyloid protein and the mechanism of Alzheimer's disease. *Trends Neurosci.*, **16** (10), 403–409.

Senin, U., Parnetti, L., Barbagallo-Sangiorgi, Bartorelli, L., Bocola, U., Capurso, A., Cuzzupoli, M., Denaro, M., Marigliano, V., Tammaro, A. E., and Fiornvanti, M. (1992) Idebenone in senile dementia of Alzheimer type: A multicentre study. *Arch. Gerontol. Geriatr.*, **15**, 249–260.

Seubert, P., Vigo-Pilfrey, C., Esch, F., Lee, M., Dovey, H., Davis, D., Sinha, S., Schlossmacher, M., Whaley, J., Swindlehurst, C., McCormack, R., Wolfert, R., Selkoe, D. J., Lieberburg, I., and Schenk, D. (1992) Isolation and quantification of soluble Alzheimer's β-peptide from biological fluids. *Nature*, **359**, 325–327.

Sheu, K.-F., Kim, Y.-T., Blass, J. P., and Weksler, M. E. (1985) An immunochemical study of the pyruvate dehydrogenase deficit in Alzheimer's disease brain. *Ann. Neurol.*, **17**, 444–449.

Shigematsu, K., and McGeer, P. L. (1992) Accumulation of amyloid precursor protein in damaged neuronal processes and microglia following intracerebral administration of aluminium salts. *Brain Res.*, **593**, 117–123.

Shioi, J. S., Anderson, J. P., Ripellino, J. A., and Robakis, N. K. (1992) Chondroitin sulfate proteoglycan form of the Alzheimer's β-amyloid precursor. *J. Biol. Chem.*, **267**, 13819–13822.

Shivers, B. D., Hilbich, C., Multhaup, G., Salbaum, M., Beyreuther, K., and Seeburg, P. H. (1988) Alzheimer's disease amyloidogenic glycoprotein: expression pattern in rat brain suggests a role in cell contact. *EMBO J.*, **7**, 1365–1370.

Shoji, M., Golde, T. E., Ghiso, J., Cheung, T. T., Estus, S., Shaffer, L. M., Cai, X-D., McKay, D. M., Tinter, R., Frangione, B., and Younkin, S. G. (1992) Production of the Alzheimer's amyloid β protein by normal proteolytic processing. *Science*, **258**, 126–129.

Siesjö, B. K., Agardh, C.-D., and Bengtsson, F. (1989) Free radicals and brain damage, *Cerebrovasc. Brain Metab. Rev.*, **1**, 165–211.

Sims, N. R., Finegan, J. M., and Blass, J. P. (1987) Mitochondrial respiratory function in brain tissue in primary degenerative dementia. *Brain Res.*, **436**, 30–38.

Sisodia, S. S. (1992) β-amyloid precursor protein cleavage by a membrane bound protease. *Proc. Natl Acad. Sci. USA*, **89**, 6075–6079.

Sisodia, S. S., Koo, E. H., Beyreuther, K., Unterbeck, A., and Price, D. L. (1990) Evidence that beta-amyloid protein in Alzheimer's disease is not derived by normal processing. *Science*, **248**, 492–495.

Smith, C. D., Carney, J. M., Starke-Reed, P. E., Oliver, C. N., Stadtman, E. R., Floyed, R. A., and Markesbery, W. R. (1991) Excess brain protein oxidation and enzyme dysfunction in normal aging and in Alzheimer disease. *Proc. Natl Acad. Sci. USA*, **88**, 10540–10543.

Smith, C. M., and Swash, M. (1978) Possible biochemical basis of memory disorder in Alzheimer's disease. *Ann. Neurol.*, **3**, 471–473.

Snow, A. D., and Malouf, A. T. (1993) *In vitro* and *in vivo* models to unravel the potential roles of β/A4 in the pathogenesis of Alzheimer's disease. *Hippocampus*, **3**, 257–268.

Sorbi, S., Bird, E. D., and Blass, J. P. (1983) Decreased pyruvate dehydrogenase complex activity in Huntington and Alzheimer brain. *Ann. Neurol.*, **24**, 72–78.

Stein-Behrens, B., Adams, K., Yeh, M., and Sapolsky, R. (1992) Failure of beta-amyloid protein fragment 25–35 to cause hippocampal damage in the rat. *Neurobiol. Aging*, **13**, 577–580.

Stephenson, D. T., Rash, K., and Clemens, J. A. (1992) Amyloid precursor protein accumulates in regions of neurodegeneration following focal cerebral ischemia in the rat. *Brain Res.*, **593**, 128–135.

Strauss, S., Bauer, J., Ganter, U., Jonas, U., Berger, M., and Volk, B. (1992) Detection of interleukin-6 and α2-macroglobulin immunoreactivity in cortex and hippocampus of Alzheimer's disease patients. *Lab. Invest.*, **66**, 223–230.

Strittmatter, W. J., Saunders, A. M., Schmechel, D., Pericak-Vance, M., Enghild, J., Salvesen, G. S., and Roses, A. D. (1993a) Apolipoprotein E: High avidity binding to β-amyloid and increased frequency of type 4 allele in late-onset familial Alzheimer's disease. *Proc Natl Acad. Sci. USA*, **90**, 1977–1981.

Strittmatter, W. J., Weisgraber, K. H., Huang, D. Y., Dong, Li-Ming, Salvesen, G. S., Pericak-Vance, M., Schmechel, D., Saunders, A. M., Goldgaber, D., and Roses, A. D. (1993b) Binding of human apolipoprotein E to synthetic amyloid β peptide: Isoform-specific effects and implications for late-onset familial Alzheimer's disease. *Proc. Natl Acad. Sci. USA*, **90**, 8098–8102.

Struble, R. G., Powers, R. E., Casanova, M. F., Kitt, C. A., Brown, E. C., and Price, D. L. (1987) Neuropeptidergic systems in plaques of Alzheimer's disease. *J. Neuropathol. Exp. Neurol.*, **46**, 567–584.

Subbarao, K. V., Richardson, J. S., and Ang, L. C. (1990) Autopsy samples of Alzheimer's cortex show increased peroxidation *in vitro. J. Neurochem.*, **55**, 342–345.

Sunderland, T., Molchan, S., Lawlor, B., Martinez, Mellow, A., Martinson, H., Putnam, K., and Lalonde, F. (1992) A strategy of 'combination chemotherapy' in Alzheimer's disease: Rationale and preliminary results with physostigmine plus deprenyl. *Int. Psychogeriatr.*, **4** (Suppl. 2), 291–309.

Tanzi, R. E., Gusella, J. F., Watkins, P. C. *et al.* (1987) Amyloid β-protein gene; cDNA, mRNA distributions and genetic linkage near the Alzheimer locus. *Science*, **325**, 880-883.

Tanzi, R. E., McClatchy, A. I., Lamperti, E. D., Villa-Kornaroff, L., Gusella, J. F., and Neve, R. L. (1988) Protease inhibitor domain encoded by an amyloid precursor mRNA associated with Alzheimer's disease. *Nature*, **331**, 528–530.

Tariot, P. N., Cohen, R. M., Sunderland, T., Newhouse, P.A., Yount, D., Mellow, A. M., Weingartner, H., Mueller, E. A., and Murphy, D. L. (1987) L-Deprenyl in Alzheimer's disease: preliminary evidence for behavioral change with monoamine oxidase B inhibition. *Arch. Gen. Psychiatry*, **44**, 427–433.

Vigo-Pilfrey, C. (1993) The role of β-amyloid peptide as a diagnostic and prognostic marker of Alzheimer's disease. Presented at Frontiers of Alzheimer's Disease. Instituto Juan March, Center for International Meetings on Biology, Madrid.

Volicer, L., and Crino, P. B. (1990) Involvement of free radicals in dementia of the Alzheimer type: A hypothesis. *Neurobiol. Aging*, **11**, 567–571.

Waite, J., Cole, G. M., Frautschy, S. A., Conner, D. J., and Thal, L. J. (1992) Solvent effects of beta protein toxicity in vivo. *Neurobiol. Aging*, **13**, 595–600.

Wakita, H., Tomimoto, H., Akiguchi, I., Ohnishi, K., Nakamura, S. and Kimura, J. (1992) Regional accumulation of amyloid β/A4 protein precursor in the gerbil brain following transient cerebral ischemia. *Neurosci. Lett.*, **146**, 135–138.

Walker, D. G., and McGeer, P. L. (1992) Complement gene expression in human brain: comparison between normal and Alzheimer disease cases. *Mol. Brain Res.*, **14**, 109–116.

Walker, D. G., and McGeer, P. L. (1993) Complement gene expression in neuroblastoma and astrocytoma cell lines of human origin. *Neurosci. Lett.*, **157**, 99–102.

Wallace, W. C., Bragin, V., Robakis, N. K., Sambamurti, K., VanderPutten, D., Merril, C. R., Davis, K. L., Santucci, A. C., and Haroutunian, V. (1991) Increased biosynthesis of Alzheimer amyloid precursor protein in the cerebral cortex of rats with lesions of the nucleus basalis of Meynert. *Mol. Brain Res.*, **10**, 173–178.

Wallace, W., Ahlers, S. T., Gotlib, J., Brain, V., Sugar, J., Bluck, R., Shea, P. A., Davis, K. L., and Haroutunian, V. (1993) Amyloid precursor protein in the cerebral cortex is rapidly and persistently induced by loss of subcortical innervation. *Proc. Natl Acad. Sci. USA*, **90**, 8712–8716.

Weidemann, A., Konig, G., Bunke, D., Fischer, P., Salbaum, J. M., Masters, C. L., and Beyreuther, K. (1989) Identification, biogenesis, and localization of precursors of Alzheimer's disease A4 amyloid protein. *Cell*, **57**, 115–126.

Weinberg, J. B., Mason, S. N., and Wortham, T. S. (1992) Inhibition of tumor necrosis factor-α (TNF-α) and interleukin-1β (IL–1β) messenger RNA (mRNA) expression in HL-60 leukemia cells by pentoxifylline and dexamethasone: dissociation of acivicin-induced TNF-α and IL-β mRNA expression from acivicin-induced monocytoid differentiation. *Blood*, **79**, 3337–3343.

Whitehouse, P. J., Price, D. L., Clark, A. W., Coyle, J. T. and DeLong, M. K. (1981) Alzheimer disease: evidence of selective loss of cholinergic neurons in the nucleus basalis. *Ann. Neurol.*, **10**, 122–126.

Wisniewski, T., Castano, E., Ghiso, J., and Frangione, B. (1993a) Cerebrospinal fluid inhibits Alzheimer β-amyloid fibril formation in vitro. *Ann. Neurol.*, **34**, 631–633.

Wisniewski, T., Golabek, A., Matsubara, E., Ghiso, J., and Frangione, B. (1993b) Apolipoprotein E: binding to soluble Alzheimer's β-amyloid. *Biochem. Biophys. Res. Commun.*, **192**, 359–365.

Yankner, B. A., and Mesulam, M.-M. (1991) β-Amyloid and the pathogenesis of Alzheimer's disease. *N. Engl. J. Med.*, **325**, 1849–1857.

Yates, C. M., Butterworth, J., Tennant, M. C., and Gordon, A. (1990) Enzyme activities in relation to pH and lactate in postmortem brain in Alzheimer-type and other dementias. *J. Neurochem.*, **55**, 1624–1630.

Yoshikai, K., Sasaki, H., Doh-ura, K., Furuya, H., and Sakaki, Y. (1990) Genomic organization of the human amyloid-protein precursor gene. *Gene*, **87**, 257–263.

Zemlan, F. P., Thienhaus, O. J., and Bosmann, H. B. (1989) Superoxide dismutase activity in Alzheimer's disease: possible mechanism for paired helical filament formation. *Brain Res.*, **476**, 160–162.

Zweig, R. M., Ross, C. A., Hedreen, J. C., Steele, C., Cardillo, J. E. *et al.* (1988) The neuropathology of aminergic nuclei in Alzheimer's disease. *Ann. Neurol.*, **24**, 233–242.

8
Multiple Neurotransmitter Strategies for Treatment of Alzheimer's Disease

F. J. Huff

Hoechst-Roussel Pharmaceuticals Inc., Somerville, New Jersey, USA

INTRODUCTION

Neurochemical studies comparing postmortem brain specimens from patients with Alzheimer's disease against specimens from age-matched non-demented individuals have revealed deficiencies in several of the classical neurotransmitters. The deficiency in acetylcholine is the most prominent among these in terms of the average magnitude across Alzheimer's disease cases, the consistency of the finding from one study to another and correlation with dementia symptoms (Davies and Maloney, 1976; Perry *et al.*, 1978; Katzman, 1986). Related to the loss of acetylcholine in the cerebral cortex is a loss of cholinergic cells in the nucleus basalis of Meynert, which projects to the cortex (Whitehouse *et al.*, 1982). Probably next in importance behind acetylcholine among neurotransmitters that are deficient in Alzheimer's disease is norepinephrine, which has been found to be depleted in cerebral cortex in numerous studies (Adolfsson *et*

Alzheimer's Disease: Clinical and Treatment Perspectives. Edited by N. R. Cutler, C. G. Gottfries and K. Siegfried.

al., 1979; Perry *et al.*, 1981; Mann *et al.*, 1982; Arai *et al.*, 1984; Rossor and Iverson, 1986). A corresponding loss of noradrenergic neurons has been documented in the locus coeruleus, which projects to the cerebral cortex (Bondareff *et al.*, 1982). A less consistent finding has been loss of brain serotonin in Alzheimer's disease. In contrast, quantities of the classical neurotransmitter dopamine have generally been found to be normal or nearly normal in Alzheimer's disease brain. In addition to these changes in classical neurotransmitters, deficiencies in peptide neurotransmitters have also been documented, the earliest of which was a deficiency of somatostatin in cerebral cortex (Davies *et al.*, 1980; Rossor *et al.*, 1980).

Treatment of Alzheimer's disease has been attempted using strategies that augment cholinergic activity in the central nervous system. The most successful among these have been acetylcholinesterase inhibitors. Tacrine (Davis *et al.*, 1992; Farlow *et al.*, 1992) and velnacrine (Cutler *et al.*, 1990; Murphy *et al.*, 1991; Siegfried, 1992) have shown modest benefit in about one third of patients as measured by the Alzheimer's Disease Assessment Scale (ADAS) (Rosen *et al.*, 1984). Although this outcome is clinically important in that it provides a treatment for at least some patients with Alzheimer's disease, it is clear that more effective treatments should be possible. A strategy toward finding such treatments is discussed below, involving simultaneous enhancement of multiple neurotransmitters documented to be deficient in patients with Alzheimer's disease. The discussion will focus on combined treatment of the acetylcholine and norepinephrine transmitter deficiencies.

ANIMAL MODELS

In developing such strategies, it is useful to have distinct animal models for the cholinergic and adrenergic deficiencies. Animal models of amnesia due to acetylcholine deficiency include blockade of muscarinic receptors using scopolamine (Shutske *et al.*, 1989), and placement of lesions in the cholinergic nucleus basalis (Haroutunian *et al.*, 1985). In both models, animals are found to be impaired in learning and memory tasks. Putative treatments may be tested by examining their capacity to reverse the memory deficits of these animals. Similarly, animal models of amnesia due to norepinephrine deficiency include blockade of synthesis by inhibition of the enzyme dopamine-beta-hydroxylase, and placement of lesions in the locus coeruleus or ascending noradrenergic bundle, resulting in deficiencies of cortical norepinephrine (Haroutunian *et al.*, 1990). Another model of adrenergic deficiency is the aged rhesus monkey, which has been shown to have a relative depletion of norepinephrine compared with younger monkeys (Arnsten and Goldman-Rakic, 1985, 1990). Potential cognitive enhancing drugs are tested for their ability to reverse the learning and memory impairment in animals with adrenergic deficiencies.

COMBINED TREATMENT WITH ALPHA-ADRENERGIC AGONISTS AND CHOLINERGIC AGENTS

A drug that has been studied as a potential treatment for adrenergic deficiency and its cognitive effects is clonidine. Clonidine is an alpha-adrenergic agonist, with a complex pharmacologic profile (Langer, 1981). Low doses of clonidine stimulate presynaptic alpha-2 receptors, resulting in a decreased release of norepinephrine at the synapse. This effect is detectable as a decrease in locus coeruleus unit firing activity in electrophysiologic studies, and a decrease in brain norepinephrine turnover through measurement of levels of the norepinephrine metabolite MHPG. At higher doses, clonidine stimulates postsynaptic alpha-2 receptors. Thus, at low doses, clonidine down-regulates adrenergic neurotransmission, whereas at higher doses it up-regulates adrenergic transmission.

The effects of clonidine on memory in adrenergic-deficient monkeys was reported by Arnsten and Goldman-Rakic (1985, 1990). Clonidine was found to improve deficits of aged monkeys on a spatial working memory task involving a delayed response paradigm, and object feature recognition on a delayed non-match-to-sample task. Clonidine also improved memory deficits of young monkeys with norepinephrine depletion resulting from 6-hydroxydopamine lesions in the dorsal lateral prefrontal cortex, supporting the specificity of the norepinephrine effect in aged monkeys. In these studies, the dose–response curves were triphasic. Both low and high doses impaired performance, whereas improvement in performance was observed in a middle dose range which varied from 0.001 to 0.08 mg/kg in different animals.

The first reported use of clonidine to treat amnesia in humans was a study by McEntee and Mair (1980). They studied eight patients with amnesia due to Korsakoff's syndrome, who were treated with 0.3 mg clonidine b.i.d. for two weeks. Improvement was observed on the Wechsler Memory Scale and a trigrams memory test. Mair and McEntee (1986) replicated this result in another eight patients with Korsakoff's syndrome, who were treated with clonidine 0.2 mg q.i.d. for two weeks, and showed improvement on Wechsler Memory Scale subtests and the trigrams test.

A study of clonidine treatment for Alzheimer's disease was reported by Mohr and colleagues (1989). They examined eight patients using doses of 0.1 to 0.4 mg of clonidine. One hypertensive patient received incremental doses up to 1.2 mg/day, administered as 0.4 mg t.i.d. They observed adverse effects at doses greater than 0.2 mg, including decreased blood pressure and mild sedation. At 0.4 mg, two patients had symptomatic hypotension. The psychometric test battery revealed no consistent effect of clonidine on attention, verbal memory, or visual-spatial memory. The authors concluded that the doses used were possibly too low to achieve cognitive effects, and increase of the dose was limited by the emergence of adverse effects.

Another attempt at adrenergic treatment of Alzheimer's disease, in combination with simultaneous cholinergic treatment, was reported by Bierer and colleagues (1993). They performed a double-blind crossover study of the alpha-2 antagonist yohimbine and the cholinesterase inhibitor physostigmine. Yohimbine was given in single doses of 10 mg or 20 mg, crossed with placebo. Concurrently, physostigmine 2 mg every 2 hours or its placebo every 2 hours were administered. In ten patients with Alzheimer's disease, no effect on the ADAS was observed comparing yohimbine or the combined treatment to placebo. A mild physostigmine effect was demonstrated by comparison with its placebo. One patient had a three hour episode of chest pain, with concurrent p-wave inversion in lead V_2, during dosing with yohimbine 10 mg and physostigmine. A myocardial infarction was excluded by serial electrocardiograms and enzyme tests. Although this study failed to reveal a treatment effect using combined cholinergic and adrenergic drugs, the conclusion is limited because only single doses of yohimbine were studied. It is possible that treatment effects would emerge during chronic dosing with an adrenergic treatment.

SINGLE AGENT WITH CHOLINESTERASE INHIBITING AND ADRENERGIC EFFECTS

A single agent with multiple neurotransmitter actions would be easier to administer than a combination of agents with different actions. One agent that has been studied in Alzheimer's disease is suronacrine (HP 128). Suronacrine is a derivative of the cholinesterase inhibitor velnacrine, in which a benzyl group has been added to the amino nitrogen (Shutske *et al.*, 1989). Suronacrine inhibits presynaptic uptake of norepinephrine, as well as inhibiting acetylcholinesterase. The compound enhances memory in rats with combined cholinergic and adrenergic lesions (Santucci *et al.*, 1991).

Suronacrine was studied in 16 patients with Alzheimer's disease who demonstrated no efficacy and no toxicity during a study of velnacrine (Huff *et al.*, 1991). Twelve patients received ascending doses of suronacrine over 6 days, followed by 100 mg b.i.d. for 4 days, and 4 patients received placebo treament. Slight improvements observed on the ADAS and a global rating in patients receiving suronacrine were not statistically distinguishable from performance in the placebo group.

One patient discontinued treatment after the first dose of 50 mg of suronacrine due to dizziness, epigastric pain, irregular pulse, and mild increase in blood pressure. Other patients experienced mild orthostatic and gastrointestinal symptoms that did not require discontinuation of treatment. Further study with higher doses of suronacrine was not pursued because plasma levels varied substantially, suggesting that in many patients tolerance would be poor at higher doses.

POTASSIUM-CHANNEL BLOCKING AGENTS WITH MULTIPLE NEUROTRANSMITTER EFFECTS

Potassium channel blockers have been examined as potential cholinergic and adrenergic treatments for Alzheimer's disease (Wiseman and Jarvik, 1991). The cholinesterase inhibitor tacrine also blocks potassium channels at relatively higher concentrations (Drukarch *et al.*, 1987), possibly contributing to its efficacy. The nonselective potassium channel blocker 4-aminopyridine is known to increase the release of acetylcholine and possibly of norepinephrine at brain synapses (Lavretsky and Jarvik, 1992). Wesseling *et al.* (1984) reported less deterioration on a rating scale and on a memory test in fourteen patients with Alzheimer's disease treated with 4-aminopyridine 10 mg b.i.d. compared to placebo for 12 weeks. Davidson *et al.* (1988) studied another fourteen patients with Alzheimer's disease. Patients were given 4-aminopyridine 2.5 mg, 5 mg, and 10 mg b.i.d. for 4 days each. The optimum dose selected for each patient was studied against placebo for 4 days in a replication crossover test. No effect on the ADAS was detectable.

Another potassium channel blocker studied in Alzheimer's disease has been linopirdine (Dup 996). Linopirdine is known to enhance the release of acetylcholine, dopamine, and serotinin (Zaczek *et al.*, 1993). Further physiological studies have revealed that the releasing effect on acetylcholine occurs only in the presence of high potassium concentrations but no effect occurs during electrical stimulation, suggesting that linopirdine may be of limited use as an acetylcholine releaser *in vivo* (Smith *et al.*, 1993).

A potassium channel blocker currently being studied for treatment of Alzheimer's disease is besipirdine (HP 749), which is an indole substituted analog of 4-aminopyridine (Cornfeldt *et al.*, 1990; Huger *et al.*, 1990; Klein *et al.*, 1991; Hubbard *et al.*, 1991). Besipirdine is a selective M-channel blocker. The M-channel is a potassium channel that is inactivated by muscarinic agonists. However, besipirdine is not a potent muscarinic or nicotinic agonist. Besipirdine is not an effective acetylcholine releaser: basal release of acetylcholine occurs only at high (millimolar) concentrations. It also is not a cholinesterase inhibitor. Evidence of an independent binding site for besipirdine has been observed, which may mediate the M-channel effect.

Physiological cholinergic effects of besipirdine have been documented. It reversed the effect of hemicholinium-3 (an acetylcholine depleter) on wave VI of the brain-stem auditory evoked potential. Besipirdine also reverses a scopolamine-induced memory deficit on passive avoidance memory in mice. Across the dose range 0.02 through 0.31 mg/kg, the optimal dose of besipirdine is 0.08 mg/kg in this paradigm. Another peak effect emerges at the 0.63 mg/kg dose, which may reflect the emergence of an adrenergic effect in these adrenergically intact animals, although this interpretation has not been directly tested.

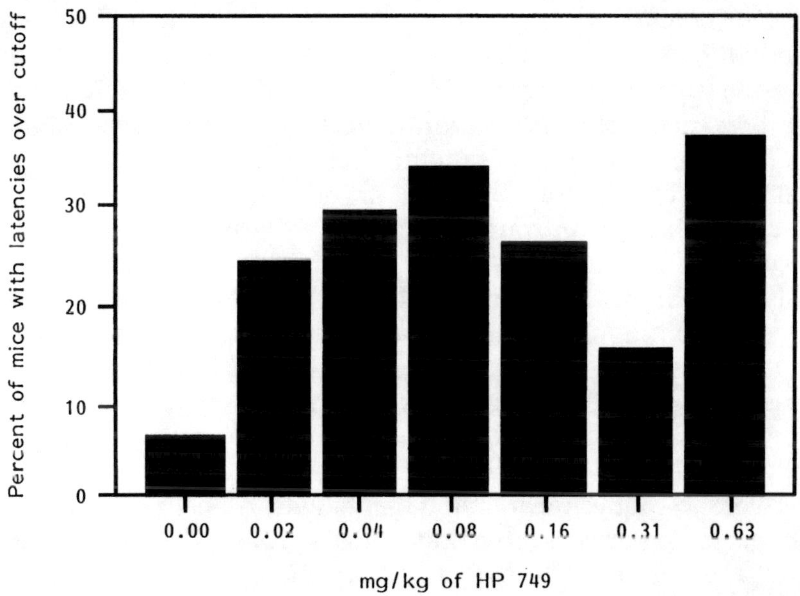

Figure 1 *Effect of besipirdine (HP 749) on scopolamine-induced amnesia in a passive dark avoidance paradigm in mice (Shutske* et al., *1989; Cornfield* et al., *1990). Scopolamine (3 mg/kg s.c.) was administered 30 min before a single training session. A dose of HP 749 or vehicle was administered 5 min prior to training. Training consisted of placement in the light compartment of a two-compartment box, and administering a 0.4 mA shock when the animal entered the dark compartment. After 24 h, animals were again placed in the light compartment, and latency to enter the dark compartment was measured. The second highest latency in the vehicle treated group was used as a cutoff to determine activity in the HP 749 dosage groups, for which results are expressed as percentage of mice with latencies over the cutoff, reflecting retention of dark avoidance from the training session*

Besipirdine has multiple adrenergic properties. It inhibits the neuronal presynaptic uptake of the monoamines norepinephrine, dopamine, and to a lesser extent serotinin. It is also an alpha-2 receptor antagonist, resulting in increased release of norepinephrine from presynaptic terminals. The *N*-dealkylated metabolite of besipirdine is itself an alpha-1 agonist and alpha-2 antagonist. Besipirdine is not a monoamine oxidase inhibitor. Probably resulting from its inhibition of monoamine uptake, besipirdine is active in a number of tests predictive of antidepressant efficacy. Doses required for efficacy in these models are higher than the doses found to be efficacious on cognitive tests. The dose range for efficacy was between 4 and 12 mg/kg on the tetrabenazine ptosis prevention test in mice, the 5-HT seizure potentiation test in rats, and the yohimbine toxicity potentiation test in mice, whereas the effective doses in the internal capsule lesion in rats were 0.31 to 0.63 mg/kg. The effective dose in the latter test overlaps with the higher peak dose in the scopolamine-dementia paradigm discussed above.

The combined cholinergic and adrenergic agonist properties of besipirdine were examined in rats with lesions in both the cholinergic nucleus basalis and the adrenergic ascending noradrenergic bundle (Santucci *et al.*, 1991). The purely cholinergic agent physostigmine is ineffective in reversing memory deficits in these animals. Besipirdine reversed a deficit in retention of passive dark avoidance at doses ranging from 0.02 to 0.08 mg/kg. The 0.08 mg/kg dose was the highest dose studied in this model, and corresponds to a human dose of about 5 mg.

Tolerance of besipirdine in patients with Alzheimer's disease has been examined in ascending doses from 5 through 60 mg b.i.d. The minimum dose for an intolerable adverse effect was 60 mg b.i.d., at which dose one of eight patients treated experienced angina. The angina resolved within hours, and a myocardial infarction was excluded by follow-up examinations. Angina is attributable to the alpha-1 agonist vasoconstrictive property of besipirdine. The maximum tolerated dose in this study was 50 mg b.i.d., at which dose one of eight patients had severe vomiting requiring discontinuation of treatment. Vomiting is attributable to the cholinergic effect of besipirdine. The dose range selected for efficacy studies is 5 to 40 mg b.i.d. Adverse effects seen in this dose range include bradycardia and postural hypotension, which are attributable to both cholinergic and adrenergic effects. The bradycardia and postural hypotension have generally been asymptomatic. A few patients have reported dizziness and lightheadedness, but this has not prevented continuation of treatment in most cases.

CONCLUSIONS

Combined cholinergic and adrenergic treatments for Alzheimer's disease have thus far produced disappointing efficacy, and tolerance factors have limited escalation of dosage in order to fully test the viability of this approach to treatment. However, a new generation of agents with multiple neurotransmitter effects manifest acceptable tolerance through the efficacy range predicted by animal models. Clinical efficacy trials are in progress for one such compound: besipirdine (HP 749). Multiple neurotransmitter strategies remain attractive for drug discovery efforts.

REFERENCES

Adolfsson, R., Gottfries, C. G., Roos, B. E., and Winblad, B. (1979) Changes in the brain catecholamines in patients with dementia of Alzheimer's type. *Br. J. Psychiatry*, **135**, 216–223.

Arai, H., Kosaka, K., and Iizuka, R. (1984) Changes of biogenic amines and their metabolites in post-mortem brains from patients with Alzheimer's-type dementia. *J. Neurochem.*, **43**, 388–393.

Arnsten, A. F. T., and Goldman-Rakic, P.S. (1985) α2-adrenergic mechanisms in prefrontal cortex associated with cognitive decline in aged nonhuman primates. *Science*, **230**, 1273–1276.

Arnsten, A. F. T., and Goldman-Rakic, P. S. (1990) Analysis of alpha-2 adrenergic agonist effects on the delayed nonmatch-to-sample performance of aged Rhesus monkeys. *Neurobiol. Aging*, **11**, 583–590.

Bierer, L. M., Aisen, P. S., Davidson, M., Ryan, T. M., Stern, R. G., Schmeidler, J., and Davis, K. L. (1993) A pilot study of oral physostigmine plus yohimbine in patients with Alzheimer's disease. *Alzheimer Dis. Assoc. Disorders*, **7**, 98–104.

Bondareff, W., Montjoy, C. Q., and Roth, M. (1982) Loss of neurons of origin of the adrenergic projection to cerebral cortex (nucleus locus ceruleus) in senile dementia. *Neurology*, **32**, 164–168.

Cornfeldt, M., Wirtz-Brugger, F., Szewczak, M., Blitzer, R., Haroutunian, V., Effland, R., Klein, J., and Smith, C. (1990) HP 749, a pharmacological profile of a therapeutic agent for Alzheimer's disease (I). *Abstr. Soc. Neurosci.*, **16**, 612.

Cutler, N. R., Murphy, M. F., Nash, R. J., Prior, P. L., and De Luna, D. M. (1990) Clinical safety, tolerance, and plasma levels of the oral anticholinesterase 1,2,3,4-tetrahydro-9-aminoacridine-1-ol-maleate (HP 029) in Alzheimer's disease: preliminary findings. *J. Clin. Pharmacol.*, **30**, 556–561.

Davidson, M., Zemishlany, Z., and Mohs, R. C. (1988) 4-Aminopyridine in the treatment of Alzheimer's disease. *Biol. Psychiatry*, **23**, 485–490.

Davies, P., and Maloney, A. J. F. (1976) Selective loss of central cholinergic neurons in Alzheimer's disease. *Lancet*, **ii**, 1403.

Davies, P., Katzman, R., and Terry, R. D. (1980) Reduced somatostatin-like-immunoreactivity in cerebral cortex from cases of Alzheimer's disease and Alzheimer's senile dementia. *Nature (Lond.)*, **288**, 279–280.

Davis, K. L., Thal, L. J., Gamzu, E. R., Davis, C. S., Woolson, R. F., Gracon, S. I., Drachman, D. A., Schneider, L. S., Whitehouse, P. J., Hoover, T. M., Morris, J. C., Kawas, C. H., Knopman, D. S., Earl, N. L., Kumar, V., Doody, R. S., and the Tacrine Collaborative Study Group (1992) A double-blind, placebo controlled multicenter study of tacrine for Alzheimer's disease. *N. Engl. J. Med.*, **327**, 1253–1259.

Drukarch, B., Kits, K. S., Van der Meer, E. G. Lodder, J. C., and Stoof, J. C. (1987) 9-amino-1,2,3,4-tetrahydeoacridine (THA), an alleged drug for the treatment of Alzheimer's disease, inhibits acetylcholinesterase and slow outward K^+ current. *Eur. J. Pharmacol.*, **141**, 153–157.

Farlow, M., Gracon, S. I., Hershey, L. A., Lewis, K. W., Sadowsky, C. H., and Dolan-Ureno, J. (1992) A controlled trial of tacrine in Alzheimer's disease. *JAMA*, **268**, 2523–2529.

Haroutunian, V., Kanof, P. D., and Davis, K. L. (1985) Pharmacological alleviation of cholinergic lesions induced memory deficits in rats. *Life Sci.*, **37**, 945–952.

Haroutunian, V., Kanof, P. D., Tsuboyama, G., and Davis, K. L. (1990) Restoration of cholinomimetic activity by clonidine in cholinergic plus noradrenergic lesioned rats. *Brain Res.*, **507**, 261–266.

Hubbard, J. W., Hsu, R. S., Griffiths, L., Dean, R., Dileo, E. M., and Hintze, T. H. (1991) The pharmacokinetics and cardiovascular pharmacodynamics of HP 749 (besipirdine hydrocholoride) and metabolite P86–7480 in the conscious monkey. *J. Clin. Pharmacol.*, **3**, 864.

Huff, F. J., Antuono, P., Murphy, M., Beyer, J., and Dobson, C. (1991) Potential clinical use of an adrenergic/cholinergic agent (HP 128) in the treatment of Alzheimer's disease. *Ann. NY Acad. Sci.*, **640**, 263–267.

Huger, F., Smith, C., Petko, W. W., Conway, P. G., Effland, R., and Klein, J. (1990) HP 749, a potential agent for the treatment of Alzheimer's disease (II): Neurochemical profile. *Abstr. Soc. Neurosci.*, **16**, 612.

Katzman, R. (1986) Alzheimer's disease. *N. Engl. J. Med.*, **314**, 964–973.

Klein, J., Davis, L., Olsen, G., Cornfeldt, M., Huger, F., Smith, C., Petko, W., Wilker, J., Blitzer, R., Landau, E., Haroutunian, V., and Effland, R. C. (1991) Synthesis and SAR of HP 749 and related analogs: Potential therapeutic agents for Alzheimer's disease. *201st National Meeting of the American Chemical Society (abstract)*, MEDI 66.

Langer, S. Z. (1981) Presynaptic regulation of the release of catecholamines. *Pharmacol. Rev.*, **32**, 337–362.

Lavretsky, E. P., and Jarvik, L. F. (1992) A group of potassium-channel blockers–acetylcholine releasers: New potentials for Alzheimer's disease? A review. *J. Clin. Psychopharmacol.*, **12**, 110–118.

Mair, R. G., and McEntee, W. J. (1986) Cognitive enhancement in Korsakoff's psychosis by clonidine: A comparison with L-Dopa and Ephedrine. *Psychopharmacology*, **88**, 374–380.

Mann, D. M. A., Yates, P. O., and Hawkes, J. (1982) The noradrenergic system in Alzheimer and multi-infarct dementias. *J. Neurol. Neurosurg. Psychiatry*, **45**, 113–119.

McEntee, W. J., and Mair, R. G. (1980) Memory enhancement in Korsakoff's psychosis by clonidine: Further evidence of a noradrenergic deficit. *Ann. Neurol.*, **27**, 466–470.

Mohr, E., Schlegel, J., Fabbrini, G., Williams, J., Mouradian, M., Mann, U. M., Claus, J. J., Fedio, P., and Chase, T. N. (1989) Clonidine treatment of Alzheimer's disease. *Arch. Neurol.*, **46**, 376–378.

Murphy, M. F., Hardiman, S. T., Nash, R., Huff, F. J., Demkovich, J. J., Dobson, C., and Knappe, U. E. (1991) Evaluation of HP 029 (velnacrine maleate) in Alzheimer's disease. *Ann. NY Acad. Sci.*, **640**, 253–262.

Perry, E. K., Tomlinson, B. E., Blessed, G., Bergmann, K., Gibson, P. H., and Perry, R. H. (1978) Correlation of cholinergic abnormalities with senile plaques and mental test scores in senile dementia. *Br. Med. J.*, **2**, 1457–1459.

Perry, E. K., Tomlinson, B. E., Blessed, G., Perry, R. H., Cross, A. J., and Crow, T. J. (1981) Neuropathological and biochemical observations on the noradrenergic system in Alzheimer's disease. *J. Neurol. Sci.*, **51**, 279–287.

Rosen, W. G., Mohs, R. C., and Davis, K. L. (1984) A new rating scale for Alzheimer's disease. *Am. J. Psychiatry*, **141**, 1356–1364.

Rossor, M., and Iversen, L. L. (1986) Non-cholinergic neurotransmitter abnormalities in Alzheimer's disease. *Br. Med. Bull.*, **42**, 70–74.

Rossor, M. N., Emson, P. C., Montjoy, C. Q., Roth, M., and Iversen, L. L. (1980) Reduced amounts of immunoreactive somatostatin in the temporal cortex in senile dementia of Alzheimer's type. *Neurosci. Lett.*, **20**, 373–377.

Santucci, A. C., Haroutunian, V., and Davis, K. L. (1991) Pharmacological alleviation of combined cholinergic/noradrenergic lesioned induced memory deficits in rats. *Clin. Neuropharmacol.*, **14**, S1–S8.

Shutske, G. M., Pierrat, F. A., Kapples, K. J., Cornfeldt, M. L., Szewczak, M. R., Huger, F. P., Bores, G. M. Haroutunian, V., and Davis, K. L. (1989) 9-amino-1,2,3,4-tetrahydroacridin-1-ols: synthesis and evaluation as a potential Alzheimer's disease therapeutic. *J. Med. Chem.*, **32**, 1805–1813.

Siegfried, K. (1992) A placebo-controlled crossover study of velnacrine in patients with Alzheimer's disease (Abstract). *Neurology*, **42** (Suppl. 3), 141.

Smith, C. P., Brougham, L. R., and Vargas, H. M. (1993) Linopirdine (DuP 996) selectively enhances acetylcholine release induced by high potassium, but not electrical stimulation, in rat brain slices and guinea pig ileum. *Drug Dev. Res.*, **29**, 262–270.

Wesseling, H., Agoston, S., Van Dam, G. B., Pasma, J., DeWitt, D. T., and Havinga, H. (1984) Effects of 4-aminopyridine in elderly patients with Alzheimer's disease. *N. Engl. J. Med.*, **310**, 988–989.

Whitehouse, P. J., price, D. L., Struble, R. G., Clark, A. W. and Coyle, J. T. (1982) Alzheimer's disease and senile dementia: loss of neurons in the basal forebrain. *Science*, **215**, 1237–1239.

Wiseman, E. J., and Jarvik, L. F. (1991) Potassium channel blockers: could they work in Alzheimer's disease. *Alzheimer Dis. Assoc. Disord.*, **5**, 25–30.

Zaczek, R., Tinker, W. J., Logue, A. R., Cain, G.A., Teleha, C. A., and Tam, S. W. (1993) Effects of linopirdine, HP 749, and glycyl-prolyl-glutamate on transmitter release and uptake. *Drug Dev. Res.*, **29**, 203–208.

9

The Use of Bridging Studies in Drug Development for Alzheimer's Disease Therapeutics

N. R. Cutler[1], J. J. Sramek[1], and M. F. Murphy[2]

[1]California Clinical Trials, Beverly Hills, CA, USA. [2]Cephalon, Inc., West Chester, PA, USA

INTRODUCTION: THE PROBLEM

A number of practical considerations have encouraged reliance on healthy normals in phase I trials, including not only medical–legal problems with patients and concerns of safety with already compromised individuals, but also convenience and tradition (Weissman, 1981). Nevertheless, where there has been strong rationale for doing so, researchers have deviated from the standard, and argued that there are persuasive reasons for utilizing patients in the early testing of a drug's safety and tolerance (Weissman, 1981; Oates, 1971). As a result, patients, not healthy volunteers, have been incorporated into phase I studies for a number of indications, including cancer, AIDS, epilepsy, and psychiatric conditions such as schizophrenia, depression, and anxiety (Cutler *et al.*, 1992c).

Alzheimer's Disease: Clinical and Treatment Perspectives. Edited by N. R. Cutler, C. G. Gottfries and K. Siegfried.

In trials of compounds for cancer and AIDS, healthy normals have been excluded for ethical reasons in view of the strong potential for adverse events (Lipsett, 1982; Spilker, 1992; Hollister, 1972). Target populations are also used in phase I studies when their presence is considered necessary for accurate pharmacokinetic evaluations—for example, subjects with epilepsy may metabolize drugs differently from normal volunteers (Spilker, 1987). This observation runs counter to the axiom suggesting that metabolic differences between normal volunteers and patients are not significant enough to support the inconvenience and potential lack of rigor associated with patient-based pharmacokinetic trials (Brazzell and Colburn, 1986). Volunteer healthy populations have also proved less useful in predicting antischizophrenic activity in compounds being developed for psychiatric patients (Gelijns, 1990). With anti-psychotic, dopamine-blocking compounds, normals have a much lower tolerability than schizophrenic patients, and thus the target population has been used in early trials in order to more accurately determine tolerated doses. In light of these facts, L. Weissman has said, 'It is not surprising that we often find ourselves requiring different doses when we move from Phase I administration in normals to Phase II treatments of patients' (Weissman, 1981).

OVERVIEW OF THE 'BRIDGING' PROTOCOL

In essence, a 'bridging study' is a late phase I evaluation, in which the patient population is utilized to help predict the safety and tolerance of the compounds being tested. By deviating from the standard clinical testing procedure and including AD patients—in addition to normal volunteers—in phase I trials under a double-blind protocol, a more thorough assessment of the safety/tolerance profile of the compounds studied is achieved while a more thorough exploration of the influence of the administration route, food/fasting and concurrent medical disorders (e.g. renal or hepatic insufficiency) proceeds in parallel (Bergstrom and Lemberger, 1990).

In studies of potential AD compounds, evaluations of healthy elderly subjects have failed to predict safety and tolerability in AD cohorts. In fact, even within the same class of compounds, widely varied responses to investigational drugs between the healthy elderly and AD subjects are observed, with both positive and negative safety implications for AD patients. Adverse events (and their severity) associated with CNS-active compounds were different in AD patients from age-matched normal volunteers (Cutler *et al.*, 1992c). The finding that safety/tolerance profiles of a compound in the healthy elderly population may be a poor indication of the expected profiles in AD patients argues for tailoring phase I studies to include the target population in a 'bridging' protocol, thus providing more valuable, more highly predictive information than can be obtained from an elderly normal cohort.

The crucial nature of obtaining such information prior to the inception of phase II trials is made clear by consideration of potential dose–response relationships (Figure 1). For the majority of CNS-active drugs, a linearity of dose and response is generally seen across both efficacy and safety variables. Indeed, clinically important organ toxicity is intrinsically linked to cumulative metabolic load. Although more complicated dose–effect relationships have been suggested for cognitive enhancers (i.e. an inverted 'U'), completed patient studies suggest that both response magnitude and frequency of response increase linearly with dosage. Because of the nature of the disease (including its pathology and the challenges of making an early, accurate diagnosis), the potential for detecting efficacy (and toxicity) in a population of AD patients thus may often exist only at the highest tolerable doses. The dose–response relationship may operationally be conceived of in terms of a 'spectrum' with no effect and no adverse events found at the end of the lower doses and strong efficacy responses but unacceptable adverse events found at the opposite end of the scale. The Maximum Tolerated Dose (MTD) with the highest potential for a significant response, will be found between these limits. Accurate definition of the MTD avoids putting patients at unnecessary risk for serious complications, while maximizing the potential for achieving efficacy. We define the MTD in relation to a Minimum Intolerated Dose (MID): the MID is that dose at which clinically unacceptable adverse events occur in a majority (≥50%) of subjects or a serious adverse event (potentially life threatening, mandating direct medical intervention) occurs in one or more subjects.

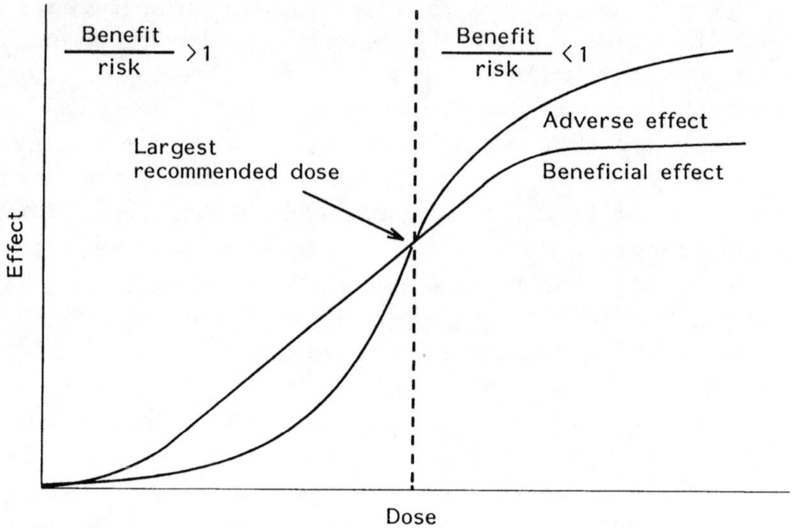

Figure 1 *The relationship between dose and effect: a risk/benefit analysis*

EVOLUTION OF THE BRIDGING STUDY CONCEPT

Initial evidence for differences in safety and tolerability between AD patients and healthy subjects was derived from 'bridging studies' with two acetylcholinesterase inhibitors—velnacrine maleate (an aminoacridine) and a carbamate derivative. As studies have suggested a cholinergic basis for the signs and symptoms of AD, the symptomatic treatment of this disease has concentrated on strategies targeting the brain's cholinergic system dysfunction.

Velnacrine Maleate

A bridging study was preceded by a single oral dose phase I study of velnacrine maleate (also known as mentane or HP029), performed in 70 young healthy male volunteers (ages 18–39) and investigating the tolerability of eight dosages: 5, 10, 25, 50, 75, 100, 150, and 200 mg (Puri *et al.*, 1989). Six subjects received active drug and three received placebo in all but two dose groups (5 mg and 100 mg); because of subject ineligibility, only five subjects received active drug in both the 5 mg and the 100 mg groups. No abnormalities were observed in vital signs, physical examination, clinical laboratory findings, or electrocardiogram (ECG). All doses, including the highest dose tested (200 mg), were considered well tolerated, and adverse events occurred in two subjects: one volunteer in the 75 mg group experienced dizziness, loose stool, vomiting and moderate headache, and one in the 200 mg cohort complained of a moderate headache. Peak plasma levels of velnacrine were reached in approximately one hour, and the drug was eliminated rapidly, with a half-life of about two hours.

A separate single-dose, double-blind, placebo-controlled, inpatient phase I study in 45 healthy elderly subjects (ages 60–83 years) evaluated the safety and tolerability of five dosages (50, 100, 150, 200, 300 mg) (Puri *et al.*, 1988). Of the nine subjects in each dose group, six received active drug and three received placebo. No clinically important drug-related changes were observed in the physical examination, ECG, or clinical laboratory findings. While no side-effects were observed in the lower dose cohorts (50, 100 mg), minor gastrointestinal symptoms were reported with dosages of 150 mg and 200 mg. All six volunteers in the highest dose group (300 mg) experienced side-effects (gastrointestinal cramps, nausea, vomiting, diarrhea), and that dosage was not considered well tolerated. Consequently, 100 mg was defined as the highest well-tolerated dose. The placebo-treated subjects reported no side-effects. Peak plasma concentrations were reached in 0.9 to 1.7 hours, and the drug was eliminated with a half-life of 2.5 to 3.1 hours.

A multiple, ascending oral dose, double-blind, placebo-controlled study of velnacrine was then conducted in 56 healthy, elderly men (mean age 67 years) (Puri *et al.*, 1990). In the inpatient study, safety and tolerability were evaluated in doses of 25, 50, or 100 mg administered twice daily (b.i.d.) or 100 mg three times daily (t.i.d.) for 28 days. Fourteen volunteers (10 on velnacrine, 4 on placebo) were enrolled in each of the four dose groups. No clinically significant adverse events were observed in these elderly men: among subjects in the 100 mg b.i.d. dose group, five on active drug experienced diarrhea, one of whom also reported nausea and another who had blood-streaked stools related to hemorrhoids; diarrhea also occurred in three volunteers in the 100 mg t.i.d. dose group. However, most of these gastrointestinal side-effects were reported during the initial nine days of dosing, did not recur, and required no treatment. There were no clinically significant or drug-related changes observed in physical examinations, ECGs or laboratory results in any of the dose levels. Peak plasma concentrations were achieved in 1.0 to 1.3 hours, and the drug was eliminated with a half-life of 1.7 to 3.1 hours. No dose above 100 mg t.i.d. was evaluated, and 100 mg t.i.d. was designated as the maximum tolerated dose (MTD). Thus, the development of velnacrine maleate followed a traditional path: studies were performed first in young and then in elderly normal volunteers, first with single doses and then with multiple doses, during which time a pharmacokinetic profile was obtained and the influence of food and fasting evaluated.

In a randomized, double-blind, placebo-controlled 'bridging study' of velnacrine, the tolerability of this compound was investigated in dosages escalating up to 450 mg/day, based on the belief that AD patients would be able to tolerate a higher dosage of a cholinomimetic than was well tolerated in the normal elderly trial (300 mg/day) (Cutler *et al.*, 1990). The rationale for evaluating this higher dosage was the assumption that the AD population would require higher dosages than normals to obtain the desired therapeutic effect, due to the documented loss of cholinergic neurons in the neocortical projection systems within the brains of AD patients, coupled with the need to increase cholinergic activity to counter the clinical deficits pathognomonic of AD (Davies and Maloney, 1976; Whitehouse, 1991).

Twenty-four AD patients (12 male, 12 female, mean age 73, range 56 to 89 years) participated in the study in a hospital setting (Cutler *et al.*, 1990). Patients were diagnosed for AD by NINCDS-ADRDA criteria, and had a mini-mental status examination (MMSE) score between 10 and 26. Patients were screened for medical, neurologic, or psychiatric illnesses or other abnormalities that might interfere with the absorption, distribution, metabolism, or excretion of the study drug.

Patients were randomized to receive either velnacrine or placebo for 10 days in a double-blind, sequential escalation study. Three groups of eight patients each were tested, with six in each group receiving the active compound. Maximum daily dosages of velnacrine were 450, 300, and 225 mg, divided into three doses per day (t.i.d.). However, poor tolerance was observed in the 450 mg/day cohort, and the group I trial was discontinued on day five. Side-effects in the 450 mg/day group included mild nausea, vomiting, abdominal cramps, dizziness, and syncope. A single clonic/tonic seizure occurred in one subject six hours following the second of three scheduled doses of 150 mg, after experiencing protracted nausea, vomiting and hyperventilation. Plasma concentrations of velnacrine were several-fold higher than those measured in normal volunteers. A protocol revision was instituted, with lower doses selected for the remaining groups.

For the remainder of the trial, groups II and III were titrated up to 300 mg/day and 225 mg/day, respectively. In the patients receiving 300 mg/day, 4 of 6 subjects on active drug were terminated from the trial early due to severe adverse effects, primarily headache and dizziness or fainting. Other adverse events in these patients included nausea and vomiting. The 300 mg/day dose was deemed tolerable in the hospital setting, but not tolerable for future outpatient efficacy trials.

The 225 mg/day dosage—25% lower than the 300 mg/day well tolerated in the earlier multiple-dose study in healthy elderly volunteers—was well tolerated in the AD patients (group III). Mild adverse events occurred in only two patients on the active drug, and included nausea, vomiting, lacrimation, and rhinorrhea, and all patients on the 225 mg/day dosage completed the trial successfully. No patients in any of the dosage groups showed any significant changes in heart rate, blood pressure, laboratory values, or ECG findings during the trial.

In summary, the velnacrine bridging study demonstrated that AD patients tolerated lower dosages of drug than both young and elderly normals. The well-tolerated dosage of 300 mg/day predicted by studies performed in healthy elderly subjects proved unacceptable in AD patients. Therefore, based upon inpatient experience with the target population, 225 mg/day was determined to be the maximum tolerated dose (MTD) in the AD population for use in multicenter outpatient trials.

In this bridging study, the importance of subject selection is apparent, in that the response of a single patient could determine the ultimate dose. Thus both the frequency and severity of the adverse event can independently influence a decision for further dose escalation. We also recognized that 300 mg may have been the MTD if the drug were given at a slower titration or for a longer duration to allow for development of tolerance. Finally, the experience provided an argument for pharmacokinetic modeling in animals or normal volunteers where other variables influencing biodisposition can be explored prior to patient exposure (e.g. gender: Bonate, 1991).

Acetylcholinesterase Inhibitor

Prior to a bridging study of this carbamate derivative, phase I safety and tolerance trials had been conducted with normal young and elderly volunteers. A single-dose, phase I study investigated 19 young healthy subjects at dosages of 4, 8, 20, and 40 mg. At the lower doses (4, 8, 20 mg), adverse events were mild and non-specific (e.g., headaches, fatigue) (Goldberg *et al.*, 1991). In the subjects receiving 40 mg, 60% experienced moderate to severe adverse events, including nausea, blurred vision, fuzziness, dizziness, symptomatic orthostatic hypotension, headache, and palpitations associated with sinus tachycardia. In this 40 mg cohort, erythrocyte (RBC) AChE inhibition reached approximately 40%.

In a subsequent single-dose trial with eight elderly subjects, dosages of 8, 20, 32, and 40 mg were tested. The lower doses (8, 20, and 32 mg) were well tolerated, but all four subjects who progressed to 40 mg experienced adverse events, including nausea, vomiting, and headaches. A dose of 32 mg was deemed the MTD.

A multiple-dose phase I study conducted with young volunteers evaluated dosages up to and including 32 mg b.i.d. and 32 mg t.i.d. (Goldberg *et al.*, 1991) Plasma drug concentrations and RBC AChE inhibition, as well as vital signs, were measured after four days of b.i.d. administration, and after four and a half days of t.i.d. administration. At the 32 mg t.i.d. dose the only adverse events reported were a number of nonspecific CNS symptoms (difficulty concentrating; vivid, dramatic dreams).

A bridging study—a multiple-dose, randomized, double-blind, placebo-controlled trial—was conducted with 20 AD patients (12 males, 8 females, age range 57–84) (Cutler *et al.*, 1992a). Subjects received a diagnosis of probable AD based on NINCDS-ADRDA and DSM-III-R criteria, and were screened for any medical, neurologic, or psychiatric disorders, or other abnormalities which could interfere with safety or tolerance assessments.

An ascending fixed-dose stage of the trial evaluated three dosages of eptastigmine (12 mg t.i.d., 20 mg t.i.d., 28 mg t.i.d. for 14 days), which were studied successively in cohorts of 4, 8 and 8 patients, respectively, with 25% of patients in each group administered placebo. None of the adverse events reported was severe enough to require withdrawal of any of the subjects. Because an MTD for the acetylcholinesterase inhibitor was not identified with this original fixed-dose panel protocol, an escalating dose phase of the study was conducted in 5 patients (2 male, 3 female; ages 72–80), with dose titration beginning at 28 mg t.i.d. and increasing by 4 mg t.i.d. every three days until 48 mg was attained on day 16. Dosages were increased again by 4 mg t.i.d. every four days to a potential maximum of 56 mg t.i.d.

In the titration phase, all subjects (both drug and placebo) experienced one or more mild to moderate adverse events during the first 15 days of treatment (dosages less than 48 mg t.i.d.). In the four subjects receiving the active drug, the most common of these adverse events were fatigue, agitation, nausea, and loose stools. One of the five patients was discontinued after the first day of treatment due to non-drug-related nervous twitches, and was replaced. The study was halted at 52 mg t.i.d. when one patient experienced severe increased urinary frequency, a severe fall and moderate bradykinesia, and another had moderate somnolence. All adverse events were transient, however, and none was observed in the ECG or other laboratory tests conducted at the end of the study.

Because the 52 mg t.i.d. dosage produced severe adverse events in two subjects, 48 mg t.i.d. was identified as the MTD for potential phase II multicenter efficacy trials. Thus, the multiple-dose MTD in AD patients was 50% higher than the single dose of 32 mg tolerated in healthy elderly subjects.

In the velnacrine and acetylcholinesterase inhibitor trials, contrasting patterns were observed in the differences between the MTD data in AD patients and the MTD in healthy elderly volunteers. Compounds within the same class can differ markedly in their structure and pharmacokinetics. Pathologic alterations in the AD brain and peripheral nervous system, including the dynamic changes related to the cholinergic deficits in these patients, is also a likely explanation for the varying sensitivity and response to these compounds.

In the acetylcholinesterase inhibitor bridging study, the combination of the fixed dose followed by the titration amendment was an inconsistent design for dose assessment. The small number of patients in the amendment portion of the study tended to limit the reliability of the findings. Also, there may not have been sufficient exposure to each dose of drug for a true safety assessment in the amendment of the study. Finally, the lack of appreciable differences in RBC acetylcholinesterase inhibition at dosages between 32 and 48 mg suggests that plasma levels of compound were in excess of those required for therapeutic efficacy. As aggressive titration and dosing can alter drug metabolism (enzyme induction and tissue penetration), the MTD dose determined in this sequence of clinical trials may have reflected aberrant biodisposition.

CONTINUED DEVELOPMENT OF THE BRIDGING STUDY

Other cholinergic compounds have been evaluated for AD using bridging studies, including the muscarinic agonist xanomeline tartrate (Sramek *et al.*, 1994). Several investigators have reported a selective reduction of muscarinic receptors in the brain of AD patients, and there are suggestions that these receptors may be critical to memory in patients with cholinergic impairment (Pearce and Potter, 1991). A bridging study was designed to examine the safety and tolerability of this potential therapeutic agent for AD.

Xanomeline Tartrate

Preclinical studies demonstrated that xanomeline tartrate can cross the blood–brain barrier and raised hopes that its high specificity to the m_1 receptor might minimize cholinergic side-effects in man. Prior to the bridging study, safety trials of xanomeline tartrate in healthy young adults did not determine a maximally tolerated dose. At the highest dose tested in a single dose trial, 150 mg, one volunteer experienced moderate nausea, while no adverse effects were observed at doses up to 75 mg b.i.d. in a multiple dose trial. A study of healthy elderly subjects reported moderate diarrhea, nausea, vomiting, diaphoresis, and hypotension at the maximally tolerated dose of 50 mg t.i.d. However, higher doses were not tested.

These data were used to establish a protocol for a bridging study—a phase I, double-blind, placebo-controlled study in 30 AD patients (13M, 17F, age range 60 to 85, mean age 73.5 years) (Sramek *et al.*, 1994). A five-panel, fixed dose design was used in this trial with the MTD in normal subjects (50 mg t.i.d.) selected as the middle panel. The lowest dose was 50% less than the normal MTD (25 mg), while the other doses were approximately 25% less (35 mg), 25% greater (60 mg), and 50% greater (75 mg) than the normal MTD. Six patients were randomized to each panel, four of whom received active drug, and two of whom were given placebo.

All patients enrolled in the trial met AD diagnostic criteria from NINCDS-ADRDA and DSM-III-R, and scored four or greater on the Modified Hachinski Ischemia Scale and between 10 and 25 on the Mini Mental Status Examination. None of the patients had a clinically significant illness that could confound the test results, and all had a diagnosis of AD.

Two of the 30 patients were withdrawn from the study early because of adverse events. One on the 60 mg t.i.d. dose had diarrhea; another receiving 75 mg t.i.d. experienced nausea and vomiting. They were discontinued on the first and second days of the study, respectively. Overall, 17 of 20 patients (85%) receiving the active drug had adverse events, which was comparable to the placebo cohort (8/10, 80%). More than 20% taking the active compound experienced diarrhea, agitation, headache, insomnia, lightheadedness, increased urinary frequency, nausea, or perspiration, while those on placebo most often reported insomnia, fatigue, agitation, flatus, and lacrimation. Three patients given active drug (35, 50, and 75 mg t.i.d. doses) experienced no adverse events. There was no significant dose proportionality in the incidence of adverse events.

As the minimum intolerated dose (MID) had not been reached within the original study design (which tested doses up to 50% greater than the MTD in healthy elderly volunteers), the protocol was amended to evaluate three additional panels at increased dosages (up to 115 mg t.i.d.). All patients successfully completed a 90 mg t.i.d. panel. Two patients experienced gastrointestinal adverse events at the 100 mg t.i.d. dose—nausea/vomiting in both subjects, diarrhea in one of them—and they were withdrawn from the trial. On the 115 mg t.i.d. panel—the highest dose tested—one patient experienced nausea/vomiting, hypotension, hypoxia, chest tightness, lethargy, hypersalivation, and diaphoresis. Since 115 mg t.i.d. was not well tolerated, 100 mg t.i.d. was defined as the MTD for xanomeline tartrate in AD patients. This dosage was 100% greater than the MTD in the healthy elderly population.

DISCUSSION: IMPLEMENTATION OF THE BRIDGING STUDY

To thoroughly assess any compound, including tolerance and safety in phase I, testing of the target patient population may provide data that healthy populations, whether young or old, cannot. Repeatedly, in tailoring protocols to incorporate the target population, safety/tolerance findings in the AD cohort have played a critical role in helping to plan the future course of investigation for that compound, including the protocols for outpatient trials in phase II. Data generated in AD patients have been more representative of phase II experience than are data in the healthy elderly. Thus, the bridging protocol in phase I has allowed the formulation of specific toxicity endpoints that mandate drug discontinuation in subsequent multicenter outpatient trials, thus protecting the target population from unnecessary risks in phase II studies (Cutler *et al.* 1992a). Since the perception of risk/benefit in AD is largely a family-driven rather than a patient-driven experience, endpoints must be operationally defined which rely on family reporting of adverse events in phase II trials. Using the findings from the velnacrine bridging study, for example, the mandatory endpoints formulated included syncope, vomiting, and severe diarrhea.

The xanomeline tartrate bridging trial illustrates the use of the fixed dose panel design to determine MTD in the target population by including the normal MTD and bracketing it at 50% less, 25% less, 25% greater, and 50% greater. The addition of higher panels when necessary to determine the MTD from the minimally intolerated dose (MID) is an integral part of the bridging protocol. In addition, to increase confidence in the MTD, the MTD panel should be repeated after the MID has been reached. This doubles the number of patients receiving the MTD dose in the phase I context and minimizes the impact of patients with idiosyncratic tolerance in an otherwise limited sample. The semi-logarithmic escalation common to phase I administration with healthy normals should be avoided in determining MTD in AD patients. Since the normal MTD has already been determined in such a manner, it is unnecessary to repeat such a dose escalation and so potentially expose the members of the target population to unnecessarily high levels of compound.

The fixed dose panel design, which requires inpatient assessment, has proven to be a valuable protocol, with advantages over slow titration in terms of maintaining safety while accurately determining the MTD. The MTD can then be used in designing dosing schedules in phase II trials, thus minimizing the risks of achieving only a 'no effect' dose in phase II (Cutler *et al.*, 1992b, 1992c). The fixed panel design neutralizes particular safety liabilities inherent in a titration protocol. First, the panel design avoids the drug accumulation (or carryover) effect which can occur in titrated dosing, thus undermining the accuracy of safety assessments in phase I. Secondly, the panel design eliminates potential problems that may occur with poor patient compliance in outpatient phase II dose titration (e.g. it predicts the effects of resuming an even larger dose of medication after missed doses).

In the titration design, there are no firm guidelines governing the rate of dose ascension. While investigators concur that the dose should be increased gradually, there is no consensus on the standard rate of escalation, or how to answer the question, 'How slow is "slow?" ' Patient tolerance varies, and a rapid titration could cause severe adverse events that can lead to cessation of the trial and even to termination of further study of a potentially useful drug. By contrast, if the dose escalation is too slow, patients may repeatedly acclimate to the compound at plasma levels which are unlikely to be tolerated through any other dose escalation scheme. If acclimatization occurs, the titration design protocol can be indefinitely extended, prolonging the clinical trial well beyond the originally planned time frame. Note, however, that higher doses of compound, regardless of titration rate, will increase metabolic load, and that metabolic load generally correlates with both the extent and type of end-organ toxicity. Without the assumption of linear dose–response relationships for efficacy, aggressive dosing to achieve a higher MTD will increase prospects for toxicity (particularly long-term toxicity) without any increase in potential benefit.

A possible alternative design combines elements of both the fixed dose and the titration designs. While the fixed dose panel could be utilized first to evaluate a compound in separate patient groups to determine the drug's MTD, a slow titration design could be employed later to move to even higher doses that would redefine the MTD in the AD population.

A bridging study could have played a valuable role in the course of drug development of tacrine (tetrahydroaminoacridine, THA), a cholinesterase inhibitor (Summers *et al.*, 1986; Davis and Mohs, 1986; Anon., 1987; Growdon, 1992). Davis *et al.* (1992), in a trial of 215 patients, concluded that although tacrine (up to 80 mg/day) produced a significantly smaller decline in cognitive function in AD patients than in a placebo group, it was not large enough to be recognized by physicians in their global evaluations of AD patients; while the tacrine group showed significantly less deterioration on the ADAS, there was no significant difference between the drug and placebo cohorts on the Clinical Global Impression of Change (CGIC). By contrast, Farlow *et al.* (1992) reported clinically significant response and reversible adverse events in 468 patients receiving similar dosages (up to 80 mg/day) of tacrine. Modest therapeutic effects in the context of acceptable risk are possible at the higher end of a presumed linear dose–response relationship. The most likely factor responsible for the underwhelming clinical effect of tacrine may be the deletion of the higher doses (120 and 160 mg/day) from the earlier completed protocols because of their propensity to cause marked liver enzyme elevations (Cutler and Sramek, 1993). Until proven otherwise, response to cholinergic replacement must be considered a linear dose-dependent phenomenon.

Although a bridging study requires careful study design and careful assessments of AD patients early in the development of a compound—and thus might lead one to argue that it is only adding an additional step to the drug evaluation process—it will ultimately result in a more efficient drug development process. In phase II trials, neither safe passage at subtherapeutic dosages nor poor tolerance and severe adverse effects because the dosages selected have been too high are desirable.

The bridging study may also be utilized for other medical indications. Earlier in this chapter, we described medical conditions (cancer, AIDS, epilepsy, psychiatric disorders) for which the target populations are already used in phase I trials, primarily for ethical reasons or to ensure accurate pharmacokinetic data. Clinical trials for other indications, such as anxiety disorders and depression—may also become good candidates for the bridging protocol.

SUMMARY

The bridging study has proven itself as a means of more thoroughly testing the potential of investigational drugs in Alzheimer's disease by incorporating target populations into phase I trials and thus optimizing safety and tolerance evaluations that can facilitate phase II and III trials. Normal volunteer studies offer convenience, methodological rigor, and systematic exploration of potential influences on biodisposition. However, extrapolation to an appropriate MTD in a patient population can be misleading, particularly if the disease presents possibilities for aberrant drug metabolism (Steventon *et al.*, 1990).

Aggressive exploration of the MTD in patients will increase prospects for toxicity but may be necessitated by compounds which have a narrow therapeutic index in a disease with few therapeutic options. In conclusion, experience with cholimimetic compounds supports the concept of a 'bridging study' as an essential component in the drug development process.

REFERENCES

Anon. (1987) Cholinergic treatment in Alzheimer's disease: encouraging results [editorial]. *Lancet*, **327**, 139–141.

Bergstrom, R. F., and Lemberger, L. (1990) First time in man studies: an industrial perspective. *J. Clin. Pharmacol.*, **30**, 212–216.

Bonate, P. L. (1991) Gender-related differences in xenobiotic metabolism. *J. Clin. Pharmacol.*, **31**, 684–690.

Brazzell, R. K., and Colburn, W. A. (1986) Controversy I: Patients or healthy volunteers for pharmacokinetic studies? *J. Clin. Pharmacol.*, **26**, 242–247.

Cutler, N. R., and Sramek, J. J. (1993) Proper development for Alzheimer's disease (letter). *N. Engl. J. Med.*, **328**, 808.

Cutler, N. R., Murphy, M. F., Nash, R. J., *et al.* (1990) Clinical safety, tolerance, and plasma levels of the oral anticholinesterase 1,2,3,4-tetrahydro-9-aminoacridin-1-ol-maleate (HP 029) in Alzheimer's disease: preliminary findings. *J. Clin. Pharmacol.*, **30**, 556–561.

Cutler, N. R., Sramek, J. J., Block, G., *et al.* (1992a) Multiple-dose safety tolerance of L-693,497 (heptylphysostigmine) in Alzheimer's disease (AD) *Biol. Psychiatry*, **31**, 155A.

Cutler, N. R., Sramek, J. J., Murphy, M. F., and Nash, R. J. (1992b) Commentary: Alzheimer's patients should be included in phase I clinical trials to evaluate compounds for Alzheimer's disease. *J. Geriatr. Psychiatry Neurol.*, **5**, 192–194.

Cutler, N. R., Sramek, J. J., Murphy, M. F., and Nash, R. J. (1992c) Implications of the study population in the early evaluation of anticholinesterase inhibitors for Alzheimer's disease (AD). *Ann. Pharmacother.*, **26**, 1118–1122.

Davies, P., and Maloney, A. J. F. (1976) Selective loss of central cholinergic neurons of the Alzheimer's type. *Lancet*, **ii**, 1403.

Davis, K., and Mohs, R. (1986) Cholinergic drugs in Alzheimer's disease. *N. Engl. J. Med.*, **315**, 1286–1287.

Davis, K. L., Thal, L. J., Gamzu, E. R., *et al.* (1992) A double-blind, placebo-controlled multicenter study of tacrine for Alzheimer's disease, *N. Engl. J. Med.*, **327**, 1253–1259.

Farlow, M., Gracon, S. I., Hershey, L. A., *et al.* (1992) A controlled trial of Tacrine in Alzheimer's disease. *JAMA*, **268**, 2523–2529.

Gelijns, A. C. (1990) *Modern Methods of Clinical Investigation.* National Academy Press, Washington, DC.

Goldberg, M. R., Barchowsky, A., McCrea, J., *et al.* (1991) Heptylphysostigmine (L-693,487): safety and cholinesterase inhibition in a placebo-controlled rising-dose healthy volunteer study, presented to: Second International Springfield Symposium on Advances in Alzheimer Therapy.

Growdon, J. H. (1992) Treatment for Alzheimer's disease? *N. Engl. J. Med.*, **327**, 1306–1308.

Hollister, L. E. (1972) Prediction of therapeutic uses of psychotherapeutic drugs from experiences with normal volunteers. *Clin. Pharmacol Ther.*, **13**, 803–808.

Lipsett, M. B. (1982) On the nature and ethics of phase I clinical trials of cancer chemotherapies. *JAMA*, **248**, 941–942.

Oates, J. A. (1972) A scientific rationale for choosing patients rather than normal subjects for phase I studies. *Clin. Pharmacol. Ther.*, **13**, 809–811.

Pearce, B. D., and Potter, L. T. (1991) Coupling of m1 muscarinic receptors to G protein in Alzheimer disease. *Alzheimer Dis. Assoc. Disord.*, **5**, 163–172.

Puri, S. K., Hsu, R., Ho, I., and Lassman, H. B. (1988) Single dose safety, tolerance and pharmacokinetics of HP 029 in healthy elderly men: a potential Alzheimer's agent. *Curr. Ther. Res.*, **44**, 766–780.

Puri, S. K., Hsu, R., Ho, I., and Lassman, H. B. (1989) Single dose safety, tolerance, and pharmacokinetics of HP 029 in young men: a potential Alzheimer's agent. *J. Clin. Pharmacol.*, **29**, 278–284.

Puri, S. K., Ho, I., and Lassman, H. B. (1990) Multiple-dose pharmacokinetics, safety and tolerance of velnacrine (HP 029) in healthy elderly subjects: a potential therapeutic agent for Alzheimer's disease. *J. Clin. Pharmacol.*, **30**, 948–955.

Spilker, B. (1987) *Guide to Planning and Managing Multiple Clinical Studies.* Raven Press, New York.

Spilker, B. (1992) *Guide to Clinical Trials.* Raven Press, New York.

Sramek, J. J., Cutler, N. R., Seifert, R. D., *et al.* (1994) The safety and tolerance of xanomeline tartrate, a M_1-specific cholinergic agonist, in patients with Alzheimer's disease. *Clin. Pharmacol. Ther.*, **55**, 174.

Steventon, G. B., Heafield, M. T. E., Sturman, S., Waring, R. H., and Williams, A. C. (1990) Xenobiotic metabolism in Alzheimer's disease. *Neurology*, **40**, 1095–1098.

Summers, W., Majoski, L., Marik, G., Tachiki, K., and Kling, A. (1986) Oral tetrahydroaminoacridine in long-term treatment of senile dementia, Alzheimer type. *N. Engl. J. Med.*, **315**, 1241–1245.

Weissman, L. (1981) Multiple-dose phase I trials—normal volunteers or patients? One viewpoint. *J. Clin. Pharmacol.*, **21**, 385–387.

Whitehouse, P. J. (1991) Pathology in the cholinergic basal forebrain: implications for treatment. *Adv. Exp. Med. Biol.*, **295**, 447–452.

Index

Note: Page references in *italics* refer to Figures; those in **bold** refer to Tables

Compiled by Annette Musker